Barbara Simonsohn

Healing Power of Papaya

**A Holistic Health Handbook on How to
Avoid Acidosis, Allergies, and Other Health Disorders**

Translated by Christine M. Grimm

LOTUS PRESS
SHANGRI-LA

The information and exercises introduced in this book have been carefully researched and passed on to the best of my knowledge and consciousness. Despite this fact, neither the author nor the publisher assume any type of liability for presumed or actual damages of any kind that might result from the direct or indirect application or use of the statements in this book. The information in this book is intended for interested readers and educational purposes.

First English Edition 2000
©by Lotus Press, Box 325
Twin Lakes, WI 53181, USA
The Shangri-La Series is published in cooperation
with Schneelöwe Verlagsberatung, Federal Republic of Germany
©1998 by Windpferd Verlagsgesellschaft mbH, Aitrang, Germany
All rights reserved
Translated by Christine M. Grimm
Cover design by Kuhn Graphik, Digitales Design, Zürich
Interior pictures: on pages 6, 135 by Dr. Garve, on page 94 by Grossmann, on pages 20, 34, 45, 68, 86, 201 by Hodapp, on page 110 by Veronika and José Perko, on page 144 by Kahuna assistant, Astara Kim Hill, on page 147 by Harald Tietze, on page 155 by Papaya John; music notes in the annex by Prost

ISBN 0-914955-63-2
Library of Congress Catalog Number 00-131343

Printed in USA

Dedication

*This book is dedicated to Ludwig Mantow,
my grandfather (104 years of age),
an example of cheerful composure,
health, and joy!*

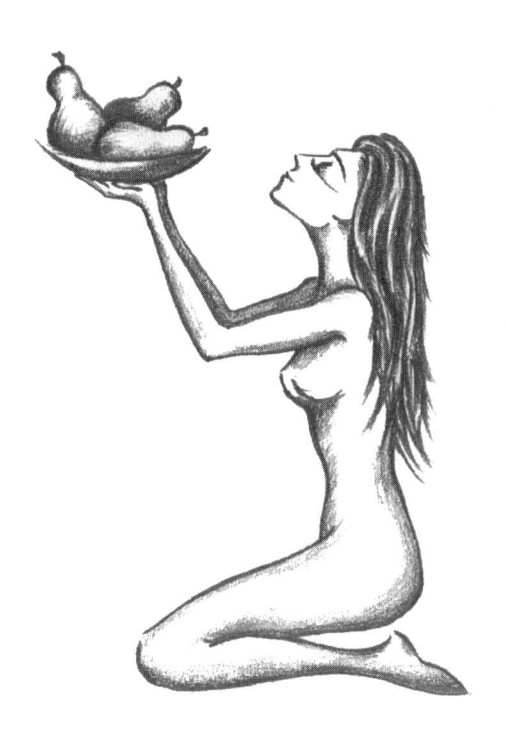

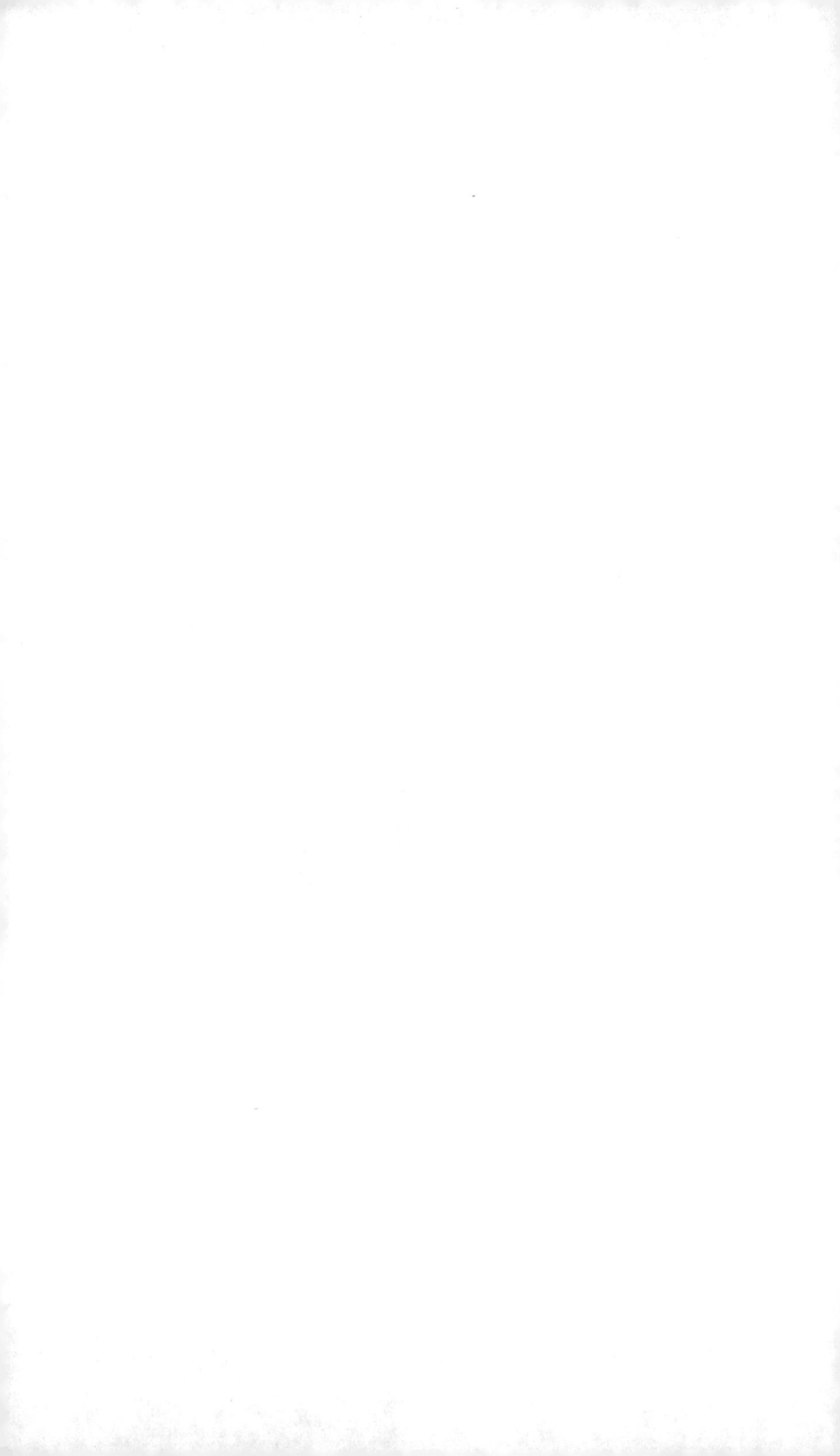

Stages

As every flower fades and as all youth departs, so life at every stage blooms in its day and may not last forever. Since life may summon us at every age, be ready, heart, for parting, new endeavors, be ready, bravely and without remorse, to find new light that old ties cannot give. In all beginnings dwells a magic force for guarding us and helping us to live. Serenely, let us move to distant places and let no sentiments of home detain us. The Cosmic Spirit seeks not to restrain us but lifts us stage by stage to wider spaces. If we accept a home of our own making, familiar habit makes for indolence. We must prepare for parting and leave-taking or else remain slaves of permanence. Even the hour of our death may send us speeding on to fresh and newer spaces, and life may summon us to newer races.

So be it, heart: bid farewell and mend!

*Hermann Hesse
(from The Glass Bead Game)*

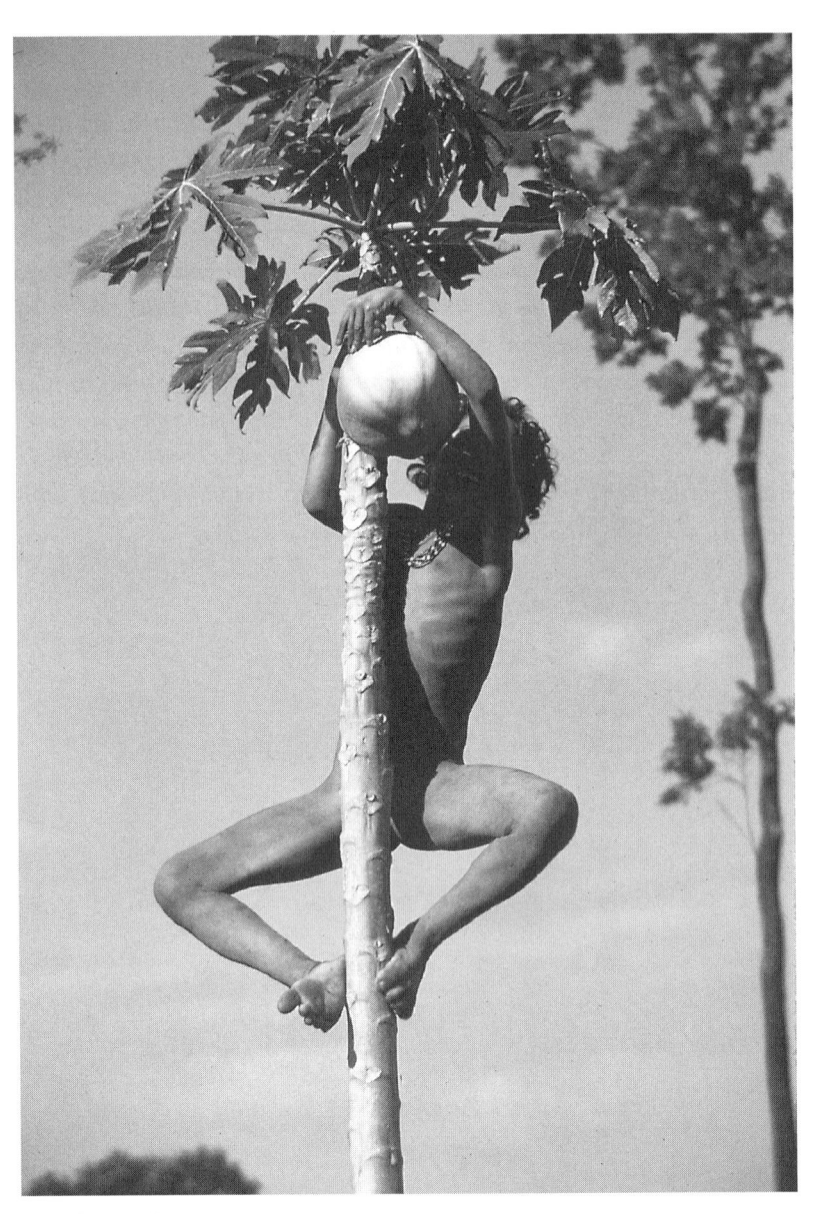

Brazil, Mato Grosso:
Boy from the Nambi Cuara picks a green papaya

Table of Contents

Dedication 3
Stages 5
Preface 11
What is Health? 13
I Take My Health in My Own Hands! 17
Sport is Suicide?—Movement is Life! 20
Emotional Health: "Stress, Get Lost!" 24
The Human Being—A Fruit-Eater? (Fruitarian) 27
Why Exotic Fruits? 30
The Papaya and I 31
The Discovery and Propagation of the Papaya 32
Can Melons Climb? 36
The Names of the Papaya 40
Organic? Naturally! 41
    Growing Your Own Papayas 42
What's in the Papaya? 46
Enzymes—The Magic Potion for Joy, Health, Beauty, and Youth 51
    Enzymes in the Papaya 53
    Enzyme Therapy 54
    Enzyme Preparations 55
Papaya Juice: A Health Cocktail 59
    Effects of Papaya Juice on Our Endocrine and Exocrine Glands 64
    Juice Recipes 66
Papaya—A Fountain of Youth 69
Papaya—Great for Sex! 71
    What Ethnologists Discovered about the Erotic Aspect of the Papaya 73
Help against Acidosis (Hyperacidity) 77
    Personal Experiences 84
Intestinal Health 87
Papaya as a Digestive Aid 91
Cancer—Causes and Alternatives 95
    Papain in Enzyme Therapy against Cancer 103
    Carpaine against Cancer? 106
    Case Example: Halima Neumann's Papaya Therapy 106

  The Papaya as Australia's Cancer-Healing "Remedy" 109

Allergies—When the "Barrel" is Full! 111
Papaya—Help for Colds and Flu 113
Papaya—Help for the Heart! 114
Papaya against Inflammation 115
Papaya Combats Fungal Disease (Mycosis) 116
Papaya Gets Rid of Worms 122
Papaya for Backaches—Chemonucleolysis and More 126
Homeopathic Applications for Papaya 130
The Papaya in Ethno-Medicine of Native Peoples 132
  The Papaya in Native Central and South American Plant Therapy 133
  The Papaya in the Folk Medicine of India 137
  The Papaya in Ayurveda—
  India's Ancient Method of Healing and Way of Life.................... 139
  The Papaya in Chinese Medicine.................................. 141
  The Papaya in Voodoo Medicine 141
  The Papaya in the Folk Medicine of Nigeria, Ghana, and Iboland 142
  The Papaya as a Healing Plant of the Kahunas, Hawaii 143
  The Papaya as a Healing Plant of the Aborigines 146
The Papaya in Beauty Care 149
Papaya John—A Life for Papayas 154
A Papaya Meditation 156
Books and Articles about Papayas 159
Recipes for the Kitchen 160
The Papaya as a Healing Remedy 167
Papaya—Healing from A to Z 173
  Additional Uses for the Papaya 198

Appendix 200
Papaya Products 202
Call for International Cooperation 203
Acknowledgments 204
The Author 206
Resources 207
Notes 208
Bibliography 211
Index 218

Papaya Hymn*

A papaya a day

A papaya a day

Keeps the doctor away

———————

Take two or three

And you will see

You will feel healthy and fine

And you will start to shine!

———————

Life gets happy as could be,

Life gets happy as could be!

---

* The music to the Papaya Hymn can be found in the Appendix

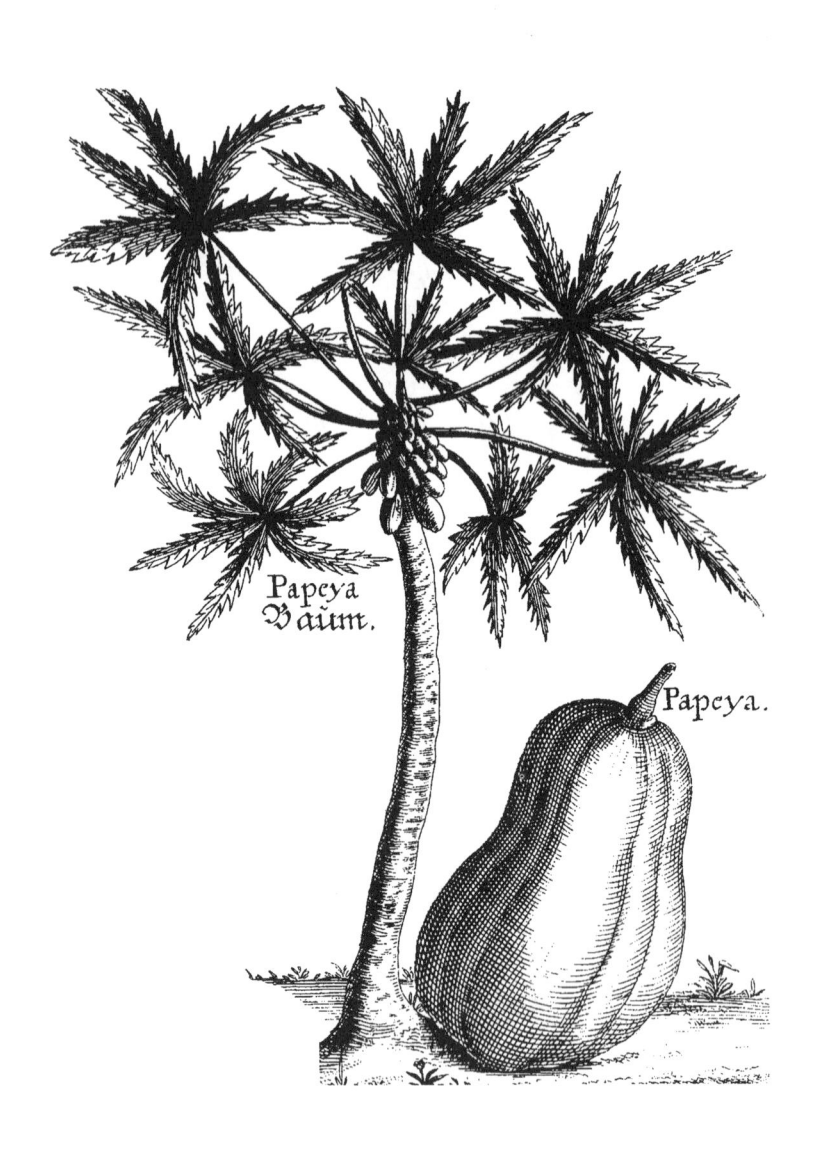

Illustration of a papaya tree with fruit from the 17th Century

Preface

Ever since I read Chester French's book, *Papaya—the Melon of Health*, I have known that Papayas not only taste wonderful but also have an extensive variety of positive effects on our health. French dedicated his entire life to research on the papaya and compiled the results in this book. As a person with a scientifically oriented approach, I was skeptical at first. "Papaya, the wonder fruit of the tropics," "tree of health," and "fruit for a long life"—I thought that this all sounded almost too good to be true!

My research has not only completely verified French's findings—it actually took my breath away! What a blessing the papaya is for maintaining our health and healing so many different complaints. Every time I thought that the papaya wouldn't have anything new to offer for a particular topic, I usually came across information a few days later confirming a related effect. When someone asks me whether the papaya might be good for a specific problem, I now say: "yes, it probably is—just give me a moment to look it up in my documentation." The enthusiasm of French and other "papaya lovers" has always proved to have a solid basis: They are not dreamers but realists!

This fruit appears to have been sent from heaven, especially for the problems that we have created because of the way we eat and live. It is really something like "the fruit of the angels," which is what the crew sailing with Christopher Columbus called it. Whether dealing with overweight, high blood pressure, arterial calcification, hyperacidity, skin problems, inflammations, varicose veins, herpes, constipation, allergies, an unbalanced intestinal flora, or infections of any kind—all of these complaints can be improved by the papaya without suppressing the symptoms. Its vital components work at the source and support the body's immune system and its other regulatory systems in functioning harmoniously. In addition, it helps to prevent illnesses before they develop. Even in difficult cases such as cancer and AIDS, the papaya presents justifiable reason for hope as both an exclusive and a supportive method of healing.

In the ethno-medicine of native peoples, the papaya has been used for these health disorders and much more since antiquity. In the

Ayurvedic way of life, it is a remedy for strengthening the life-supporting mental powers—the Sattva energy—and bringing our constitutional type into harmony. The wonderful power of the papaya is not restricted to physical health: We can become even more beautiful with it, enter into contact with our Higher Self, improve our love life, and brighten our mood.

The papaya and this book are an invitation to reconnect ourselves with Mother Nature and the nature within us, seeking the solution to our problems with her instead of fighting against her. They are also an invitation to question our lives and determine how we can attune it to natural laws, life-giving forces, and genuine values. The papaya can make it easier to abstain from many unnecessary and unwholesome things, allowing us to enjoy a healthier way of life. The wonder of the papaya is not described exhaustively in this book. Every day I receive faxes from all over the world with new application possibilities. The spectrum of application ranges from an antibiotic to a fungicide and from a virus-killer to an anti-cancer remedy.

Consequently, as the "Swiss army knife" of natural healing remedies because of its great diversity of applications, the papaya is perhaps superior to the well-known grapefruit seed extract. And just like the grapefruit seed extract, the papaya has no side effects. We will certainly still learn many new things about the papaya in the future. My appeal to you is: Try out the wonder that the papaya also offers your life and treasure the miracle of this wonder!

Barbara Simonsohn, February, 1998

What is Health?

*"Health isn't everything,
but without health everything is nothing"*

(Arthur Schopenhauer)

*Health cannot be bought -
We fight for it by changing our lives!*

(Henry Ford)

Health is something precious, the magic word of our age. Who doesn't want to be healthy, fit, and productive? Only when we are healthy, can we fully enjoy and master our lives. No wonder that health is always one of the main desires mentioned when people are surveyed.

Health is more than the absence of illness, just as peace is more than the absence of war. The World Health Organization (WHO) defines health as "feeling completely well on all levels." This also includes the social level. According to their estimates, only two percent of the world population is really healthy, a vanishingly small portion, in the sense of this definition.

We shouldn't succumb to the temptation of claiming that we are healthy just because we are not sick. Being healthy means waking up in the morning and wanting to hug the whole world! It means being constantly full of joy, curiosity, and excess energy so that after a fulfilled, happy life one can simply fall asleep. We have almost become accustomed to people dying of illness instead of just being weakened by old age. But "normal" doesn't mean "natural." We should become increasingly aware of this difference and orient ourselves toward being "natural" instead of accepting what has now become the "normal" state of illness.

Dr. Norman W. Walker, my great role model, fell asleep peacefully when he was 116 years of age. Until the very end, he rode a bicycle and wrote the last of his many books at 113.

Together with its 1997 World Health Report, the World Health Organization submitted a document about "a world-wide tragedy of suffering." WHO expects a doubling of cancer for most nations within the next 25 years! It explains the underdeveloped countries' strong increase in chronic illnesses as primarily because they have adopted unhealthy Western lifestyles. These include unbalanced nutrition with a trend toward instant meals and junk food, a lack of physical exercise, as well as tobacco and alcohol consumption. The WHO experts assume that in the threshold countries the number of deaths because of cancer and cardiovascular diseases will constantly increase. Although the life expectancy will also rise, the quality of life will sink dramatically. And isn't health expectancy more significant than life expectancy?

Many people are no longer healthy, even if they consider themselves to be. A lack of vitality, weak concentration, insufficient motivation, exhaustion, headaches, depressive moods, sleep disturbances, frequent colds, and allergies are signs that we are no longer really healthy. Are we healthy if we are always (or repeatedly) dependent upon medications and other medical help?

The truth is uncomfortable: We cannot buy health, and each of us must actively take our health into our own hands. Every moment of our lives we decide between health and life or illness and infirmity: in what foods we choose, deciding how much we exercise, whether we smoke cigarettes or drink alcohol, when and how much we sleep, and whether we allow ourselves breaks to regenerate and reduce stress.

This book should help us free ourselves from the restraints of the health-insurance system and take the responsibility for our own well-being. Correct nutrition plays a very important role in this process. More than 50 percent of health disorders leading to death are due to an improper diet! Eating too much food and the wrong food is suicide in the long run. Just as we make sure that our car has the right gas and regular oil changes, we should give our own "heart-engine" or "liver-factory" high-quality fuel, a break once in a while, and support the elimination of waste so that our body doesn't begin to "stutter" and "suddenly" come to a standstill.

Beauty and health are related. When we become healthier on the basis of a natural lifestyle, we will also become more beautiful. Our skin will be clearer, our muscles tauter, and we will radiate an enjoyment of life. Genuine health is an excess of energy and makes us attractive to others.

We are a unity of body, mind, and soul. When negative feelings are bottled up inside of us, we get upset about every insignificant incident and neglect our own personal development. When this happens, even the healthiest food won't make us completely well again. In my first two (German-language) books about the Five Tibetan Rites for Children and Authentic Reiki, as well as at my seminars, I have described in detail how we can nourish our soul correctly, decrease stress effectively, and relax deeply at any time. On the other hand, when our body is burdened with waste products and we are physically hyperacidic, we turn "sour" psychologically. Or we become depressive and non-receptive to spiritual experiences. Whenever I cannot make any progress with Reiki on a person, an acidosis treatment and long-term alteration of diet has often had a miraculous effect. This does not mean "either-or" thinking, but developing a holistic perspective and a "both-and" treatment!

Don't be seduced by the illusion of eating only pills instead of fruit and vegetables in their original state. Many of the treasures in fresh fruits and vegetables—such as bioactive substances, enzymes, and vitamins—have not yet been researched and their optimal interactions remain a puzzle. Possibilities of protecting ourselves against illness through correct nutrition are far from exhausted. Even papaya enzymes aren't the tools to repair an unhealthy lifestyle. We can't go on smoking, eating too much fat, getting inadequate physical exercise, and drinking excessive quantities of alcohol and then expect antioxidants, bioactive substances, and enzymes in the form of pills to work wonders on our health.

If we really want to protect ourselves effectively against oxidative stress and chronic illness, there is no way around a healthier lifestyle. For twenty years now, I have been a vegetarian with no milk products or eggs, eating almost exclusively raw food. I feel fit, healthy, and capable. During the eighteen years in which I have worked full-time, holding seminars and teaching Reiki almost every weekend, I have not been forced to cancel a single lecture or seminar because of illness. I nursed one of my children for 18 months and the other for two-and-a-half years. I require very little sleep (six hours). I can do a great deal, express my creativity, and have good powers of endurance. Weight problems are a thing of the past: With raw food and fresh juice, I have no difficulty maintaining my ideal weight of 130 pounds at a height of 5 feet 8 inches.

With a diet emphasizing fruit and vegetables, primarily large amounts of raw foods, we consume fewer calories, less cancer-causing matter, and less animal fat. In addition, we obtain the vital substances that we need. In this way we comprehensively protect ourselves against metabolic illnesses and effortlessly meet the American Departments of Agriculture and Health's daily requirements of at least five portions of fresh vegetables and two to five portions of fresh fruit for health care and cancer prevention.

After you have read this book, you will know that the papaya is a "wonder plant" because comprehensively affects our metabolic processes, restores health to our intestines, and can even rejuvenate the body's cells. Many of its secrets and gifts are just waiting to be discovered and put to use! The papaya is a great help during the transition to a more natural and healthier lifestyle. It facilitates and accelerates this change.

To me, the papaya is an exotic messenger from a climate where the cradle of humanity originated. With it, we can put a small piece of paradise on our plates.

I Take My Health in My Own Hands!

"People beg for health from the gods, but they don't know that they can influence it themselves" (Heraclitus, about 550 to 480 B.C.)

It's important that we assume responsibility for our own physical, emotional, and mental health. How often do I see people visit a therapist, Reiki teacher, or spiritual healer—instead of going to a physician like they used to—with the expectation of being made healthy again?

A man with lung problems, who stank of cigarettes and coughed so badly he could scarcely manage the stairs to the first floor, never returned after his first Reiki treatment: I had dared to tell him that he had to give up smoking to be cured. The consumer and pill-taking mentality has even invaded so-called "alternative medicine." When doctors or therapists recommend a radical *("radix"* means "root") change in the patient's lifestyle and eating habits, they usually meet with a long face, opposition, and often the patient stops coming.

In ancient China, doctors were paid to keep their patients healthy. When they had too many sick patients, they were warned; when the situation didn't improve, they had to find a new location for their practice. In the worst case, they were forced to give up their profession. The more patients *("patiere"* means "suffer" in Latin) our doctors and therapists have, the better off they are. We can honestly ask ourselves: Do we expect our health to be guaranteed when we pay our health-insurance bills? Today there are health insurances that pay for naturopathic treatment. As a result of this offer, the health insurance companies expect to gain new members. Is this the solution—to turn to naturopathic practitioners instead of orthodox medicine in the future?

In my opinion, the reply of "it doesn't matter if I get sick, the naturopathic doctor or healing practitioner will take care of it" is also an attitude based on consumerism. Since this mental program no longer applies to me, I have drawn the necessary conclusion: I left my health-insurance plan with the awareness that it was a final step since probably no insurance will want me when I'm older. As far as health insurance go, I am now totally responsible for myself. When I go to the dentist for a check-up every year, I pay the bill myself. When I want to have colon hydrotherapy—a thorough intestinal cleansing (see *Intestinal Health* on page 87) —I also pay the bill. This is easy for me to finance because I no longer must pay $450 per month for health insurance. Another alternative would be an inexpensive insurance with a high deductible since accidents would also be covered in this case.

Since I have a very healthy diet—almost exclusively raw foods (often from my own garden), wild herbs, sprouts, freshly squeezed juices, and no animal protein—and engage in sports every day, fast for about ten days once a year, and practice meditative techniques (Authentic Reiki) to reduce stress, I feel deeply relaxed and my emotions are harmonious. I feel like I am on the safe side: I do everything I can to maintain my health.

This radical step of doing without extensive health insurance can't be recommended to everyone since it is only advisable for those who have already concerned themselves with the topics of health and nutrition for years, practicing much of what they have learned in their daily lives. I have meditated for almost 20 years, been a vegetarian for 20 years, and have eaten almost exclusively raw plant foods for the past 12 years! I have gone through numerous healing and cleansing crises, but there will always be additional ways of positively influencing my health. It is important to remain open to real learning and attempt to increasingly translate theory into practice, without having to be perfect at it.

This greatly strengthens our self-confidence and we believe ourselves capable of even more! This year I learned to plant an elevated vegetable bed so that I can harvest most vegetables organically and fresh from my own garden. I also started a small fruit grove (hopefully a richer harvest from the frost-resistant mountain papayas will be possible in the near future!) and discovered new wild herbs—such as tasty stinging nettle seeds—to eat with exotic fruits like the papaya. I also began jogging every day. Two years ago, I discovered the power of barley grass and AFA algae, and now enjoy their strengthening effect on my nerves and brain. I have already written books (in German) about these topics!

"In all beginnings dwells a magic force." Don't be impatient with yourself, but begin—at best, today—taking your health into your own hands! Start with a papaya for breakfast, a daily walk in nature, and then slowly start reducing your addictions to substances like coffee and sugar. Perhaps you might try listening to a relaxing cassette or meditate. This is the beauty of the topic of holistic health: It doesn't matter where we begin, we will always profit from it! Since we are a unity of body, mind, and soul, everything that we do for ourselves on one level also has a positive effect on the others. If you eat more fruit, you will develop more joy in life; when you meditate, you find your way back to your acid-alkali equilibrium. As it says in the Bible: "If you take one step in the direction of God, He will run ten in your direction!"

There are an abundance of suggestions as to what this first step might be in this book. If we turn to Mother Nature or God, they will support us more and more. However, we must (or are permitted to) take the first step ourselves. I wish you much joy in doing so!

Sport is Suicide?— Movement is Life!

*"We should always remember that
our old age is the result of our earlier life
and that we harvest in old age
what we sowed in our youth and middle years."*

(Goethe)

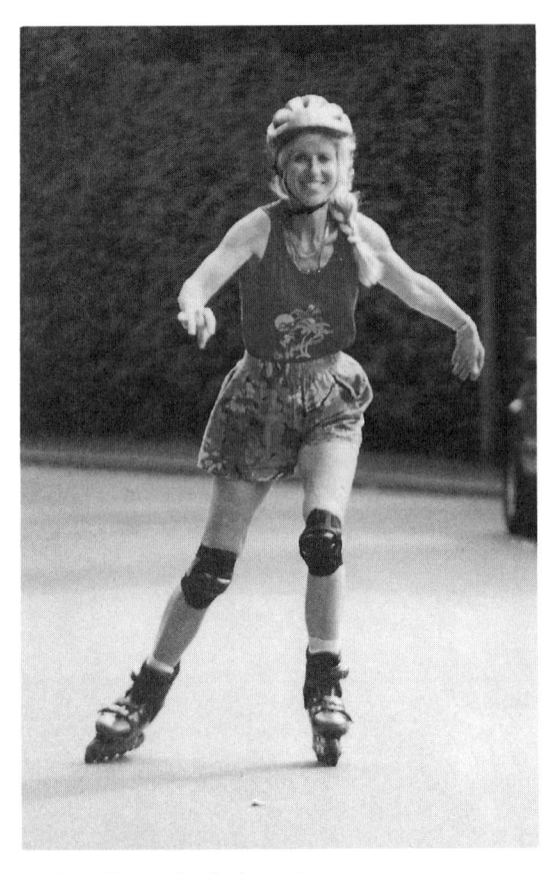

Barbara Simonsohn: body moving

There is more to health than proper nutrition. My grandfather reached the age of 104. He has maintained his mental and physical fitness—lives alone, speculates on the stock market, works in his large garden and harvests much fresh food from it, has a cheerful disposition, and gets much exercise in the fresh air. His good example shows me that "aging" doesn't have to be accompanied by complaints and infirmity!

Muscles and joints suffer from signs of wear when they have not been challenged by sports for years. The development of osteoporosis is facilitated when women do not exercise. If you stay fit, you do a great deal for the health of your heart, circulatory system, respiration, and metabolism. Even the brain enjoys improved circulation when you take a walk in nature. Sport is said to prevent Alzheimer's disease. We have more emotional endurance, reduce our level of stress, and release the "feel-good" hormones—endorphins! Through intensive exercise, the stress hormone adrenaline is broken down more quickly. "You can see this effect in the mirror immediately after training: the facial features appear much softer and more relaxed."[1]

Physical exercise is also important for our supply of enzymes: We can stimulate the production of our own enzymes, supply them to our brain and support health, joy and productivity. In addition, endurance sports protect us against "free radicals," which destroy our cells and can lead to serious diseases such as cancer. If you get your body moving on a regular basis, you will have a positive, long-term effect: "The body reacts to exercise with a lasting reduction of the pulse frequency, reduction of the blood pressure and lower-blood fat values."[2]

When I began with endurance training, my pulse was 70 beats per minute at rest. After a month, it was only 52! That's more than 25,000 beats less every day, and 9 million beats in a year. If you let your heart work in this economical way, you will get more out of it—including a longer life. "Desk workers" especially need physical exercise so that they can relax after work and maintain a state of inner balance.

The famous sports physician Professor Wildor Hollmann of Cologne commented on the massive loss of physical abilities due to lack of exercise in older people: "Normally, a person is fit for life when he is born. Only through the extreme lack of exercise in our modern lifestyle do we lose this state of fitness."[3] The German author Dr. Klaus Hoffmann notes in his book about rheumatism that there is frequently a connection between lack of exercise and spinal column disorders. For him "no illnesses are caused by wear."

The good news: It is never too late to begin with sport activities! If you start with regular exercise training like slow jogging at the age of 60, you can win back the capabilities of a 40-year-old within 10 weeks! Sport physicians have discovered that a daily training of ten minutes is more effective than an hour once a week. However, the optimum amount of activity lasts for half an hour or a whole hour per day and is so intense that you perspire.

"Become like the little children": Accept their example! They are always in motion and don't attempt to avoid it like many adults do. They always seek possibilities to be physically active. Our new sofa was immediately used by my two-year-old daughter as a trampoline and she climbs up the steep slide on the playground countless times.

The body profits most from endurance sports like gymnastics, hiking, jogging, swimming, bicycling, or cross-country skiing. Oxygen metabolism remains elevated for 24 hours after a bicycle tour or a long run, for example. Fat-reducing enzymes remain active for up to 12 hours after physical training. If you want to lose weight or remain as slender as you already are without effort, you only need to exercise regularly and eat raw food as often as possible. Another benefit is the reduction of stress resulting in a brighter mood and stronger nerves, which is also important. I jog half an hour a day, in all kinds of wind and weather. If you would rather exercise inside when the weather is bad, you can run on a miniature trampoline. When I run, I have the most creative ideas for my work or problems that need to be solved. I enjoy nature and feel fresher, happier and more balanced the entire day. It's nice to begin the day with a sense of success: I have once again conquered my "inner laziness"!

German author Franz Konz has observed "the primeval movements" of our relatives, the apes, carefully and described them in detail together with illustrations in his raw-food classic. Through these movements, our glands are activated, our cells optimally nourished, and waste is removed more quickly via the lymph flow. Dr. Edwin Flatto describes in his book *Super Potency at Any Age* how we can prevent and heal illness. For acute health disorders, rest is necessary; chronic illness requires movement! From arthritis to varicose veins to constipation, a great variety of problems can be corrected in this manner.

I "swear by" my daily Five Tibetan Rites, which uniquely strengthen muscles and glands, balancing and stimulating our energy centers. Last summer, a woman at the swimming pool asked me what fitness studio I go to because my muscles are so beautiful and my body is so well-trained. I credit my appearance mainly to the Five Tibetan Rites and secondly to jogging and garden work—despite the fact that I have inherited weak connective tissue from both sides of my family. In comparison to women my age who are less active in terms of sports, I don't have a trace of varicose veins at the age of 46!

Jogging shoes with good elasticity and shock absorption are important when running. At the beginning it may be hard to start participating in sports. After about two weeks, the "dead point" is usually overcome. Running becomes easy, you feel like a "perpetual mobile" and have the time to perceive and appreciate the beauty of nature.

Through exercise and proper nutrition, we can also reduce backaches! We need to eat many fresh foods and drink plenty of water in order to better supply our cells and remove waste materials from the body. We can support our intervertebral disks by doing body exercises that stretch and bend our spinal column. The disks suck up water like a sponge. I do one or two series of the Five Tibetan Rites every day. The exercises last only 15 minutes, but have a positive effect on my body and soul for many hours! Although I was born with a bent spine, I have no problems if I do these exercises regularly. When a doctor sees my back, he throws up his hands and thinks I must constantly be in pain!

Here's another exercise for relieving and increasing the blood flow of the disks: Lay on your stomach and place three thick pillows under the upper thigh and three pillows under the chest so that the stomach hangs down, which improves the circulation of the spine in this position.

Emotional Health: "Stress, Get Lost!"

*"Courage lost, all is forlorn,
It would be better if he hadn't been born!"*

(Goethe)

We are a unity of body, mind, and soul. We "nourish" ourselves not only from what lies on our plates, but also from vibrations. When we feel "sour" about someone or something, we also become physically acidic. When our body is too strongly acidic because of false nutrition and an improper lifestyle (also see *Help against Acidosis* on page 77), we are incapable of developing joy and love. Or, as Norman Walker, author of many wonderful books on natural health, explains with respect to intestinal health: Very few people understand how directly the condition of the large intestine is related to states of weakness, particularly stress and nervousness. He writes that it is almost impossible to keep a clear mind and maintain proper emotional and mental equilibrium when we have long neglected our intestine.[4]

Only in a healthy body can there be a healthy mind. The reverse is also true: A sick soul can make the body sick in the long run.

The more than 5000-year-old teaching of Ayurveda points out that negative feelings such as anger, rage, or envy poison our body. When fears are suppressed, kidney disorders result. Anger influences the liver while avarice and greed have a negative effect on the heart and spleen. Suppressed feelings cause disturbances in the Tridoshas, the basic constitutional characters of human beings: Suppressed fears create a Vata disturbance, anger an excess of Pita, and envy, greed, and apprehension intensify Kapha. "These imbalances of the *tridosha* affect natural body resistance (the immune system—*agni)* and thus the body becomes susceptible to disease."[5]

When Agni, the body's immune reaction is weakened, allergies to certain substances like pollen or dust can result. For this reason, the science of Ayurveda teaches that each individual must let go of such feelings.

How should we deal with our feelings according to Ayurveda? "The Ayurvedic technique for dealing with negativity is: observation and release. For example, when anger appears, one should be completely aware of it; watch this feeling as it unfolds from beginning to end. From this observation, one can learn about the nature of the anger and then let the anger go, release it."[6]

We can also approach other negative feelings in this way.

The school of Natural Hygiene places particular emphasis on "emotional hygiene."

Norman Walker proposes to watch your soul thoroughly, to study one's mood and to learn to control one's thoughts. He moreover suggests to guard one's thoughts and to decide on what thoughts may enter the mind. The reason is, towards Walker: when something has entered our mind, we tend to think about it. He stresses that we are co-creators in designing our lifes in what we see, hear, read, feel, and think. He says, on the other hand, that we have to purify our bodies in order to create a nice home for our souls. And, in the same time, we have to nourish our bodies with high-quality food that may rejuvenate and regenerate our cells and tissues.[7] In this holistic approach to health, Walker has a successful follower, David Wolfe in his phantastic and inspiring bestseller rawfood book "Sunfood Diet Success System".

Harvey and Marilyn Diamond in "Fit for Life I and II" also not only advocate a raw food diet, but also have "22 essential rules." These include happiness, love and understanding, relaxation, a feeling of belonging together, avoiding excitement, eliminating excess stress, a feeling of security in life, a joyful environment, self-mastery, useful and creative work, motivation, inspiration, contentment, self-respect, self-confidence, and a sense of self-worth. All of these requirements cannot be filled immediately, but if you make an effort and don't lose sight of this goal, you will eventually succeed.

The larger social context also plays a role in health: Fry feels that we can become emotionally balanced or happy when we know that our work is appreciated by society. We can only achieve true contentment in a society that fulfills this condition.[8]

Within this context, I recommend that you don't just wait for things to turn out all right on their own if you are unemployed or dissatisfied with your present work. You could attempt to become self-employed. If at all possible, make your hobby into your new profession. Perhaps you might even be able to make ends meet by being employed on a part-time basis and growing your own fruits and vegetables in the remaining time. You could also gather wild herbs if you live out in the country—a very satisfying occupation, I think.

For more than 18 years now, Authentic Reiki has given me the best experiences for transforming negative feelings, reducing stress, cultivating emotional contentment, relaxing deeply, and enjoying a cheerful sense of peace and tranquillity. This ancient technique for harmonizing feelings and activating the immune system is easy to learn, even for children, and works for everyone. I have successfully taught Authentic Reiki to thousands of people in Germany, in the USA, and other countries. It is a method for helping yourself, as well as others.

Learning the Five Tibetan Rites is also helpful for reducing stress and cultivating a cheerful sense of peace and joy in life. As opposed to Authentic Reiki, you can learn these exercises on your own from the book *Ancient Secret of the Fountain of Youth* by Peter Kelder.

I found a wonderful holistic statement on the topic body, mind, and soul in *The Healing Power of Grapefruit Seed,* with which I would like to close this chapter: "If we want to eliminate illness in a fundamental and lasting manner, we should start on the different levels. Measures on the mental and emotional level such as relaxation, letting go of fears, and accepting our deeper needs should be accompanied by cleansing and purifying the body from damaging microorganisms and avoiding new toxins."[9]

The Human Being—A Fruit-Eater? (Fruitarian)

Many people think that we are omnivorous by nature and proud of the fact that they "tolerate" everything. The unfortunate error regarding nutrition is that we often are not presented the "bill" in the form of lost abilities and illness until many decades later. What if we really aren't omnivorous and are actually vegetarians? Scientists believe that millions of years ago we nourished ourselves primarily from fruits. The primates that genetically resemble us most closely—their genotypes supposedly have a 98-percent correlation with our own—eat raw plant foods almost exclusively. When they have fruit available to them, they prefer it to everything else: fruit appears to be their favorite food.

The representatives of Natural Hygiene claims that our digestive system adapted itself during the course of an enormous span of time to a diet consisting of fruits. From the length of our digestive channel and shape of our teeth, it's clear that we are not meant to be meat-eaters. On the other hand, fruit is attractive to both young and old. Just the thought of a cool, ripe watermelon makes our mouth water on a hot day. Why do we instinctively long for fruit? The Diamonds assert that this is because fruit is undoubtedly the most important food, the food to which the human body has adapted in terms of its own biology.[10]

By studying the fossil teeth of our ancestors, Dr. Alan Walker, the famous anthropologist at John Hopkins University, has determined that all of the teeth studied from people who lived from 12 million years ago up to Homo erectus were the teeth of fruit-eaters—without exception.[11]

What **advantages** does fruit have? Why should we begin to view it as a basic food instead of just a snack?
- Fruit has the highest water content of all foods: between 80 and 90 percent of the best purifying water. When we eat fruit we eliminate waste substances from the body.
- Fruit contains an abundance of vitamins, minerals, carbohydrates, enzymes, amino acids, fatty acids and other bioactive substances that our body needs to live.

- Fruit requires less energy for its digestion than any other type of food. We save energy that can be put to good use for physical and mental activity by eating fruit!
- Fruit supplies our brain with the ample amount of glucose that it needs to function.
- The energy that we save through fruit is used by the body to cleanse itself and eliminate wastes, helping us to achieve our ideal weight.

However, fruit should be eaten alone or before other foods (with a twenty-minute pause) so there is no "collision" with foods that are more difficult to digest and require a longer time in the stomach. According to the Diamonds, fruit eaten in the correct manner has the wonderfully rejuvenating ability of counteracting possible excess acids in the body[12] (also see *Help against Acidosis* on page 77). Rules for eating fruit correctly can be also found in the books written by Steven Arlin and David Wolfe on the rawfood diet.

Is it possible that we originally ate mainly fruits before we were forced by external influences to change our diet? Wouldn't you like to see how you feel if you eat only fruit and drink freshly squeezed juice at least until lunch? Instead of interrupting the body's cleansing and eliminatory phase with an opulent breakfast and wasting energy on digestion, we can let the body remain free and clear. This makes us feel productive and charged with energy. We have gained energy instead of expending it.

I don't expect you to believe this, but I would like to invite you to try it out once for yourself! Eat only fruit—regardless of which kind and how much—until lunch. However, it is best if you always eat only one type of fruit at a time until you are satiated by it. Then your body has the least digestive work to do. If you keep your customary diet and follow only this piece of advice, you will quickly notice the positive effect on your health and well-being, losing any excess weight without effort. Two older women told me that they overcame their pain—one had rheumatism and the other arthritis—after following this rule for five days.

Fruit contains everything that we need. There are people in the best of health who have eaten only fruit for years, sometimes only one type of fruit. Eating sweet fruits is not only important for our body's health. The system of Ayurvedic healing and living, the oldest existing health system in the world, tells us that sweet fruits are the best diet for developing Sattva, the consciousness of light, clarity, and knowledge.

In his book on Ayurvedic cooking, Harish Johari writes that when we attain the Sattva consciousness, there is no longer anything that we need to do: We have no reason to move, no task to solve, no need for food or sleep, and no confusion in our minds. We feel bliss and joy in the state of Sattva consciousness.[13]

Each of us can bring more light into our life. We can feel lighter and more energetic. Eating the sweet fruits of paradise is a way of giving your soul more harmony and gradually merging it with the "one consciousness": Sat-Chit-Anand, truth-being-joy, will be the reward. An increase in Sattva energy and spiritual development can be supported by a Sattva diet. Johari believes that a diet consisting only of fruits such as sweet oranges, apples, bananas, grapes, and juicy mangoes is ideal.[14]

By fasting with just fruit, you can reduce your weight by an average of twelve pounds per week depending on your initial weight: If you are considerably overweight, you will lose even more. The high water and fiber content in papayas, pineapples, and mangoes stimulates elimination. In contrast to total fasting cures without any food, none of the feared health crises occur. But the results are more than just the loss of weight: The skin, intestines, and entire metabolism profit from eating a diet of just fruit. In addition, change occurs on additional levels: people become more balanced, peaceful, cheerful, and energetic.

Professor Arnold Ehret, one of the representatives of Natural Hygiene speaks from his own experience when he writes: "On the basis of my years of experimenting, I have no doubt that fruit, even just one kind of fruit, not only heals the body but nourishes it perfectly. They completely prevent illness! The more you become free of waste substances and toxins, the more sensitive your senses will become. The 'paradise fruit diet' brings you closer and closer to a physical and mental condition that you wouldn't have considered possible before!"[15] Professor Ehret, who was given up by the doctors because of a severe illness, ate only fruit for two years. Then, at the age of 39, after seven days of fasting followed by just two pounds of cherries as his only daily meal, he went on a 56-hour march through northern Italy without a break and food, but with some water, and concluded it by doing 360 knee bends—in front of witnesses!

Guy-Claude Burger, the French founder of the Instinctive Raw-Food Therapy, advocates fruits as the main food. "They represent 68 percent of the chimpanzees' food in nature, and instinct also leads humans to about this percentage."[16] Burger responded to the question of how to solve the hunger problems in Third World countries: "If people would respect primeval laws in their nutrition, this problem could be easily solved. If you love fruit, you love trees. Then you would take care of your own fruit garden. If the people in this world would think more about fruit, we could imagine how areas that are now subject to intensive agricultural exploitation are planted with thousands of types of fruit trees so that in spring a single garden would spread before us, full of flowers and fragrances..."[17]

Why Exotic Fruits?

Why do most young children usually prefer sweet bananas, mangos, or papayas to apples? Why do many adults prefer exotic fruits to those of their homeland? Burger explained it this in this way: "Today we live in latitudes to which we are not genetically adapted. It has been scientifically proved that we haven't always lived in the temperate zones. We inherited our genetic constitution from primates and they come from the tropical regions."[18] This aspect is particularly important with respect to illness: "If one has a therapeutic aim in mind, then it is good to have the broadest possible range (of fruits) available."[19] To return to our banana example: "The fact that tropical fruits taste better also shows that our organism needs the corresponding components, that they simply correspond better to our genetic constitution."[20]

I once spent two weeks in Burger's "Instincto Center" eating tropical organic fruits. I felt like I was in heaven there! At Christmas, I will order a durian fruit from Burger's tropical organic-fruit catalog as a special treat. Their fragrance and taste are simply like "paradise on earth".

The Papaya and I

After a 24-hour flight from Hamburg to Maui, Hawaii by way of Vancouver with the accompanying time change, I felt exhausted. I slept and dozed for half the day. The next morning, I still felt tired and unmotivated. The attractive surroundings left me cold and, in addition, my digestive system wasn't functioning as usual. With my fiancée, I went shopping at a natural food store in Paia. I was surprised to see cans of dried papaya seeds there. "That's funny," I thought, "there are so many papayas here. Why do the people in Hawaii throw the seeds away only to then buy them later at an expensive price in a health-food store as a digestive aid?"

We bought a few ripe papayas, and my fiancée was almost shocked to see me eat the fruit complete with skin, seeds, and stem. "That's not how you eat a papaya," he scolded while wrinkling his nose and shaking his head. "Why not?" I responded because the sharp seeds tasted pleasantly spicy together with the sweet fruit.

Immediately after eating the papaya, I felt physically and emotionally better. I was once again in a good mood and ready for adventure! Less than half an hour later, my digestive system was functioning well again.

At that time, I didn't know that the papaya has a strongly alkali-forming effect and can serve as a "mood brightener" (see *Help against Acidosis* on page 77). I was simply surprised by the prompt response as a digestive aid (see *Papaya as a Digestive Aid* on page 91).

After this key experience, I ate a papaya for breakfast whenever possible and kept this good habit even after I returned to Germany. It was only several years later that I read about the advantages of this exotic fruit and heard phrases like "a papaya a day, keeps the doctor away" or "papaya, the melon of health." As I read about the discovery of the papaya, it became clear to me that it took centuries for scientists to become interested in this fruit and explain the sensational effect of the fruit on the tormented stomachs of the Spanish conquerors.

Many "wonders" that this fruit contains have not yet been discovered and we can expect many positive surprises in the future. For example, the research on all the enzymes and other active substances is far from complete. Sometimes we need many impulses before we get enthusiastic about something.

This book is meant to encourage you in experiencing this "wonder fruit from the tropics" yourself. Fortunately, there are good habits as well as bad habits that we can establish. Perhaps the papaya will also become indispensable to your daily range of foods. The best thing about the papaya is that it not only is healthy, but also tastes fantastic!

In this sense, this book would like to arouse your appetite for this "fruit of the angels" and bring a small piece of tropical "paradise" into your home.

The Discovery and Propagation of the Papaya

The papaya plant originated in the tropics of the Western Hemisphere, in southern Mexico and Central America. It was first mentioned in 1519 in reports of the capture of Mexico by Hernando Cortez (later the Spanish conquistador in Mexico).

After a friendly welcome, Cortez destroyed the Aztec kingdom between 1519 and 1521 with the help of the Tlaxcaltecs, one of the few tribes that was independent of the Aztecs. The capital city of Tenochtitlan (today part of Mexico City) was conquered and destroyed on August 13, 1521.

The Aztecs made it easy for Cortez to conquer them since the date of the Spanish arrival corresponded with an old prophecy that the venerable Toltecan cultural hero Quetzalcoatl would return from the east, white-skinned and bearded, to ascend to the Aztec throne. This prophecy led to disaster for the Aztecs. The warrior folk saw its world threatened and destined for destruction. Their minds were filled with fear at the prophesied return of the priest king from the east, who was to put an end to the reign that demanded human sacrifice in horrible quantities for the bloody gods.

The Aztec King Montezuma II believed the Spanish were the prophesied new masters from the east and that he had to relinquish his throne to them. Cortez, who was received as a god, seized Montezuma II without a battle. Later, the Spaniards under Cortez marched further south to the Yucatan Peninsula to fight the Mayas. This major civilization had already split into small states that fought against each other, destroying their highly developed culture. Cortez crushed the Mayas in battles between 1527 and 1546 after years of embittered resistance on the Yucatan Peninsula.

Bishop Jimenez, who accompanied Cortez, provided precise documentation of the entire expedition. He wrote: "We were greeted on the shore by the Aztec chiefs as we landed and they were apparently deeply impressed by the thought of a god with red hair, blue eyes and light skin. The entire crew was majestically served many courses of the local food, until our soldiers developed problems caused by the gluttony. When the chiefs noticed this, they called their servants to bring something that was apparently a melon with golden flesh and soft skin, as large as the head of a man. They ate this fruit themselves and pressured us to do the same. In a moment our digestive problems disappeared, as if we had eaten very little."[21]

Quite astonished, the Spaniards asked to see the "wonder plant" that brought forth such fruit. When they asked its name they understood "ababai," from which they created the Spanish name "papaya." It was not until a few centuries later, at the end of the 19th century, that German scientists were the first to begin scientifically researching the effect of papayas.

There are reports that the papaya was first discovered by Marco Polo (1254-1324) in the Orient and that Vasco da Gama (1469-1524) wrote about it. These claims are false, the papaya could not have reached the Orient at this early point in time. It is suspected that these first conquerors meant the durian fruit, which is related to the papaya and also contains proteolytic (protein-splitting) enzymes, but is native to Malaysia.

Shortly after discovering the Americas, Columbus is said to have become acquainted with the papaya. His companions called it the "fruit of the angels." The Indians in tropical America valued it so highly that they ate a piece of papaya after every meal. A man from the crew reportedly told the Pope of that time that eating papaya quickly eliminated the sick feeling after the consumption of heavy, rich foods and alcoholic drinks.

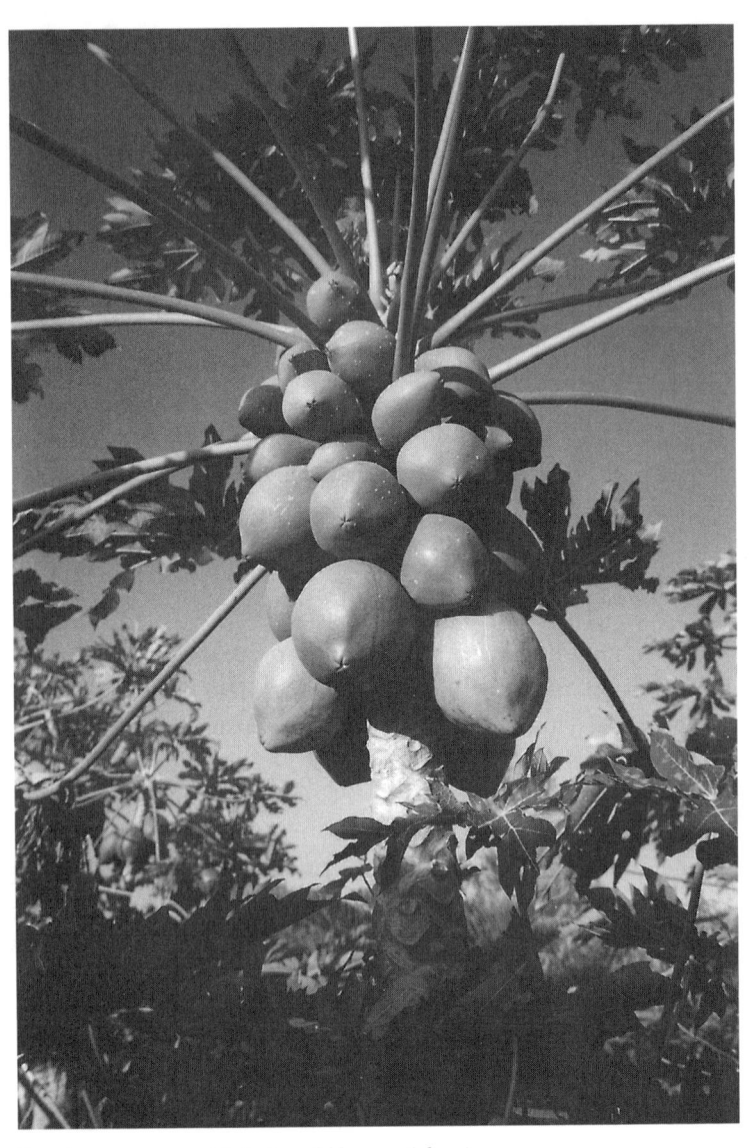

Female papaya tree with fruit and blossoms (above)

Another story tells of how the papaya was propagated: Captain James Cook brought papaya seeds back with him from Central America on his third trip seeking a northern passage from the Pacific to the Atlantic (1776-1779). He finally landed on the Kona coast of the "Big Island," where he had a skirmish with the native Kanakas. They killed him in a battle on February 14, 1779. His ship remained in the harbor for a longer period of time and social contacts developed between the soldiers and the natives. During this stay, the seeds were planted and the papaya spread from Hawaii to all of the Pacific islands.

At the beginning of the sixteenth century, Spanish soldiers brought the papaya seeds to the Philippines, from where they spread to the Orient and on to the East Indian islands. Moslems brought them from Sri Lanka (once called Ceylon) to East Africa. From here they went to Zaire, which was the Congo at the beginning of this century.

From their land of origin, Mexico, papayas were also brought to Cuba and Jamaica. Today they can be found in all subtropical and tropical regions between twenty-degrees longitude North and twenty-degrees longitude South. It's worth noting that papaya cultivation is now much more prevalent outside of Latin America than on the continent where they originated.

The papaya is cultivated primarily to obtain papain, the enzyme from the milk juice of the unripe fruit. The demand for papain has constantly risen throughout the entire world, totaling more than 300 tons a year in the USA and Europe alone.

Can Melons Climb?

"The papaya is a garden wonder."
(Sharon Tylor Herbst, "The Food Lovers Companion")

"Can melons climb?" was the title a Bern newspaper gave to an article about papayas. Although the German name means "melon tree," the papaya (botanical name: *Carica papaya*) is actually not related to the melon but to the fig *("Carica"* means fig in Latin) and passion flower (Latin: *"passifloraceae"*).

Originally a native wild plant in the marshy lowlands and coastal forests of Central America and Brazil, the papaya was spread throughout the entire tropics and subtropics by the Spaniards and Portuguese. About 50 different types are now being cultivated throughout the world. In Europe, it can be found in the Mediterranean and on the Canary Islands. The genuine wild varieties can still be found on the American continent from Mexico in the north to the subtropical valleys of Chile in the south. In Paraguay, papaya grows wild everywhere, although it was never planted as a fruit tree. The inhabitants simply tear out the excessive plants.

The most popular varieties are "Castanhal Para" from Brazil, "Sunrise" and "Sunset" from Hawaii, "Hortus Gold" from South Africa, "Betty" from Florida, and "Graham" from Mexico. The most important type in world trade is the "Solo," cultivated in Hawaii. This is a small, one-pound fruit with hardly any seeds.

If you should have the rare luck of finding a large papaya outside its native region, like Mexican papayas, you should buy it: They taste deliciously aromatic and are seldom imported because of their sensitivity to pressure.

Papayas with deep-orange flesh taste best. An example of a very tasty variety is the "Bahia" from Brazil, which might become as successful as "Solo." The former weighs about two pounds and its salmon-colored fruit flesh tastes delicious (connoisseurs say like raspberries and apricots at the same time). This exceptional taste stems from the relatively high content of fruit acid, which is often lacking in other types and makes the "Bahia" especially fruity and refreshing in comparison. With the sweet variety called "Golden Papaya," Brazil is attempting to conquer further portions of the market.

The papaya can be considered to be a "blooming biological wonder." At the end of a non-branched stem that is three to seven meters (10 to 23 feet) tall, there is a tuft of large, hand-shaped, divided leaves. They give the papaya tree—which actually is a bush from a botanical point of view—the appearance of a palm from a distance. When the leaves fall, they leave a noticeable scar on the stem. Yellow-white flowers of one-half inch to two inches in length grow from the rachis bud and smell pleasantly sweet like lily-of-the-valley. The papaya is generally dioecious, which means that female and male flowers do not occur on the same plant. When papayas are cultivated, one male plant is included for every approx. 25 female plants so that there will be good fructification.

The female flowers are larger than the male flowers and have a five-toothed calyx and a funnel-shaped corolla with five slits but no stamina. In contrast, the male flowers have ten stamina as well as a five-petal, funnel-shaped corolla with numerous branched panicles. Pollination occurs at night via hummingbirds or butterflies.

Since various tropical birds eat papaya fruit and spread the seeds, the plant can grow wild in the jungle. It often "sleeps" underground for years until a clearing develops. Then, papayas suddenly grow everywhere.

Occasionally, hermaphrodite flowers occur. In terms of botany, the papaya is also a special plant because sex changes are possible. The changing sexual conditions of *Carica* have not yet been satisfactorily explained. Indians attempt to influence these changes with the help of mystical objects such as iron nails or copper rings, which they nail into the stem. The author Chester French observed that the deeper the top soil, the more of the desired feminine species were found.

After pollination, clusters of up to twelve pounds of yellow, oval or pear-shaped "giant berries" ripen, resembling melons. From a botanical viewpoint, these are berries. The fruit has a length of about 1 foot and width of 1/2 foot, pointed at the top. The largest papayas, *Lechosas* from Venezuela, can be up to 3 feet long and are hollow inside. The fruit's form resembles the full breast of a woman. The Cubans call it *fruta de bomba* because of the similarity to a bomb.

The yellow-orange, soft, sweet and juicy fruit flesh with its butter-like consistency (but fat-free!) has a firm skin that is green on the unripe fruit and green and yellow on the ripe fruit. There are hundreds of pepper-sized, shiny black seeds that smell like cress at the center of each fruit. They taste pungent because of the mustard oils that they contain. The fruit smells somewhat like a muskmelon. The fruit flesh is largely free of acid and has a pleasantly delicious taste. Some papaya fans say the taste is somewhere between raspberry, strawberry, and cantaloupe, but it is unique.

When cultivated, papaya plants grow very quickly and may reach a height of up to 32 feet. They already bear fruit after just nine to twelve months. Because of their rapid growth and fertility, they are also viewed as a "garden wonder". After about three years, the stem is already about one foot thick and full of fruit at the top. Milk tubes pass through the plant, secreting a white milky juice when they are injured. The plants only live for about ten years. Their productivity decreases after the second year, which is why they are often replaced after the third year when cultivated.

The papaya belongs to the most common tropical trees of the tropics and subtropics. Together with bananas and cassavas, they are often grown by small farmers and are even used as feed for pigs. Plantations yield an acre harvest of about 20 tons per year. The raw material for papain (a proteolytic enzyme) is obtained by scratching the unripe fruit in the early morning hours. Despite this "milking" of the fruit, it remains suitable for consumption; however, because of the scars on the skin, it cannot be exported. Throughout the world, the papaya is primarily cultivated for papain production and only secondarily as an eating fruit. Yet, the demand for papayas in countries like the USA, Japan, and Europe is increasing strongly.

In the West Indies and other tropical islands, meat is wrapped in papaya leaves to make it tender or tough meat is rubbed with slices of green papaya, which is then cooked together with it for the meal. Papain is used today as a meat-tenderizer, particularly in the USA. In other countries like Germany, the use of papain as a tenderizer is prohibited in order to prevent customers from "being deceived." After a papain treatment, meat that had been as hard as leather becomes as tender as that of a young animal. If papain is used for too long, the meat decays. In the USA, animals are even sprayed with papain shortly before they are killed in order to make the meat more tender.

Papain is also used in tanning to make leather and soften fur, as well as for the manufacture of non-shrinking wool and silk. Except in places like Germany, where purity regulations prevent additives, papain is also used to clear beer.

The papaya loves volcanic soil. It needs protection from the wind and moderately moist soil, but is otherwise quite adaptable. However, when cultivated conventionally in mono-cultures without humus management, the papaya may be attacked by viruses and other pests (also see *Organic? Naturally!* on page 41).

At the University of Honolulu on Hawaii, a virus-resistant papaya has been developed through gene manipulation, one of the first useful plants subjected to this questionable process (I got this information from the Internet under "Papaya"). I hope that gene-manipulated fruits won't become a major export of other papaya lands as well.

An alternative to gene-manipulated plants is the development of virus-resistant wild types such as "*Carica stipulata*" and "*Carica pubescens*" by classical selective methods as well as production of illness-resistant plants under organic cultivation (also see *Organic? Naturally!* on page 41).

In the meantime, the papaya is cultivated worldwide in frost-free areas. There are organic farms in Belize (formerly British Honduras), Hawaii, Sri Lanka, Thailand, and the Canary Islands, which export organically cultivated fruits without manufactured fertilizer, pesticides, fungicides, or insecticides. Because of the small demand for exotic organic fruits, the prices are still very high.

I hope that this book helps increase the demand for organic papayas so that they can be found at the markets as a rule rather than an exception. Organically grown fruit and vegetables have a considerably higher value for our health and therapeutic purposes than the conventional products. For example, they can be used as cancer therapy (see *Cancer—Causes and Alternatives* on page 95 and *Organic? Naturally!* on page 41).

Through further propagation of cold-resistant, mountain papayas from the Andes and the increased development of the greenhouse effect, the papaya might eventually also conquer the moderate climate zones and become adapted to more northerly gardens.

The Names of the Papaya

Linneaus, a famous Swedish biologist, gave the papaya the Latin name of *Carica papaya* in 1753. *Ababai* or *mabai* means melon tree in the Caribbean language. The Mexican Indians named the papaya *ambapaya*.

In Cuba, the fruit is called *fruta de bomba* because of its shape. The British called it melon tree or *papaw* the first time that they saw it in the West Indies. The name *pawpaw* is still used in New Zealand and Australia. Another similarly named small bush or tree, the pawpaw, with small, good-tasting fruits that isn't related to the papaya, grows in the southern states of the USA. (The botanical name of this type of pineapple is *Asimina triloba* or *Annona triloba*.)

In Puerto Rico, the papaya is called *lechosa* because of the milky white juice it gives when unripe. In French-speaking lands, the names papaya, *papayier*, or *abre de mélon* are used. In Brazil, one says *mamai, mamao, mamaveria*, or *mam(a)oeira*, as well as *mamaya* in some places. It is also called *mamao* in Portugal because the fruit is reminiscent of a woman's breast. In the German-language region, the papaya used to be called *Papai, Papaya, Papaiabaum*, or *Melonenbaum* (melon tree). *Papaya* is now the most common term here as well.

Here are a few further names from various lands: *du du* in Vietnam; *malakor, ma-la-ko*, or *ma kuai the* in Thailand; *gedang* in Indonesia; in the Philippines, *papaya, kapaya*, or *lapaya*; in Burma *thimbaw*; in Cambodia *ihong* or *doeum lahong*; in Laos *houng*. The Kahunas in Hawaii call the papaya *mikana*; the Hindus in India call it *papitá* and the Tamils of southern India *pappali*. In the East Indies, the papaya is called *papayo* and in China *fan-yayzu*. There it is primarily found on the island of Haynan.

Organic? Naturally!

"Healthy soil, healthy plants, healthy people!"

"Soil fertility is the basis of all life."

(Hans Peter Rusch)

All specialists who deal extensively with the topic of human nutrition come to the conclusion that the ideal plant foods comes from organic cultivation. In large-scale industrial gardens and horticultural establishments, plants are sprayed with pesticides, fungicides, and insecticides; the growth of the plants is artificially "spiked" with industrial fertilizers. There are rising complaints that our soil is increasingly leached and our food contains less and less vitamins and minerals. There is an excellent fundamental book in German by Hans Peter Rusch about why only soil with intact soil organisms can grow healthy plants, and these in turn contribute to the human health.

The parallel behavior between infertile "dead" soil and unfruitful plants and animals cannot be disproved. The biological capacity of the soil is a prerequisite for the existence of higher life. Plant diseases and "pests," as well as the development of more and more new viruses, indicate a lack of health. Rusch considers illness and pests as the "regulators of primeval nature." A healthy soil is able to heal virus diseases, as is a healthy human organism.

Rusch goes so far as to say "one healthy apple has much more significance for our health than many poisoned apples."[22] The German physician Max Gerson sees an even greater correlation between the health of plants and the health of human beings: he considers the soil and everything that grows in it to be our external metabolism. Like Rusch, he understands the German concept of "mother soil" (topsoil) to be literal. He compares the soil with a mother nursing her child[23] and also concludes that most disease germs in a healthy soil, which is normally rich in antiviral substances, do not last very long.[24] Since Gerson recognizes that we must care for the soil so that it can produce healthy plants, he serves organically grown fruits and vegetables to his cancer patients, many of whom had been given up upon by the medical establishment. He states that when we grow foods in this way, we must eat them as living substances, as fresh as possible and prepare them immediately after they have been harvested: "Life produces life". Food from organic cultivation appears to be the solution to the cancer problem.[25]

Consequently, we should attempt to buy as much organically cultivated fruit and vegetables as possible and begin to grow them yourself. Start thinking organically and grasp the wonder that there are more living organisms in one single shovel of soil than there are people on the earth. If all modern methods of classical bacteriology were applied, without exaggeration, the study of one single soil sample would be more than a life task.[26] Organically cultivated papayas are available in stores with organic products and from mail-order companies, as well as at some weekly farmers markets. "Once you understand that every agricultural change in biological substance circulation causes damages to the substances themselves, you are forced to demand that such practices be abolished."[27]

Each of us can begin at home: I have sacrificed a piece of lawn for an elevated vegetable bed, a fruit grove, and a compost heap, where I feed the soil organisms with cut grass and weeds. Let us help a "new age of the living" to be born: "There are forces everywhere that are concerned with the full essence of living beings and not just with the measurable, countable, and weighable part."[28]

Growing Your Own Papayas

If you have a greenhouse that can be heated in winter or live in a frost-free area, you can simply take seeds from the fruit that can be purchased at the store or market. After three to six weeks, you will see the first little plants. If you don't have a greenhouse and live in a cooler climate, you should obtain the seeds or bush of a robust species that is not sensitive to the cold: the *Carica Pentagona* or the *Carica Goudotiana*, a mountain papaya that comes from Columbia and grows in the Andes at heights of up to 2,800 meters above sea level (bush about $30).

I ordered a *Carica pentagona (Babaco)* as a tub plant in a container about 90 centimeters high. This species is closely related to the well-known papaya bush and cultivated in Australia and New Zealand. It is currently "conquering" Europe because it has a pleasant taste like pineapple, strawberries and lemon. In contrast to the *Carica papaya*, it has no seeds and can be eaten completely without any waste. However, a gardener in La Palma said that they taste more like a vegetable and don't come close to the usual papaya. My *Babaco* is on the south side of our house and already has blossoms in May. Even if the fruit doesn't grow to be large enough, you can still use the leaves and stems for papaya tea.

In any case I will attempt to get my robust, mountain papayas from Columbia through the German winter. Harald Tietze, a non-fiction author living in Australia, told me that papayas are cultivated there in mountainous regions where it snows in winter. Unfortunately, the growth period is too short for them to bear fruit. However, the leaves can be used for tea. In winter, plastic bags are placed over the papaya plants to protect them.

Growing tropical fruit in colder climates should be viewed as a "hobby." If you only want to save money in comparison to buying the fruit, the high heating costs and uncertain yield will probably disappoint you. Yet, despite this, it is a thrilling and fulfilling hobby. Your own papayas will certainly taste much better than those bought at the store.

When raised in the optimal conditions of their native lands, the plants bloom and bear fruit after nine months.

When planning a greenhouse, it is important to take into consideration that papayas can grow to be eighteen feet tall and may stand six to twelve feet high when they first blossom. The papaya species that can be obtained in stores everywhere, *Carica papaya*, grows best at temperatures of 56 to 66 degrees Fahrenheit in winter. They also need a bright environment that is not too cool (lowest temperature about 52 degrees Fahrenheit). They should be watered less in winter so that the roots remain just slightly moist. The water for this purpose should be warmed beforehand. Even in winter they can be lightly fertilized every four weeks. The *Carica papaya* on the Canary Islands only grows in areas up to 650 feet above sea level because it is very sensitive to the cold. I sent seeds from the cold-resistant Andes papaya to a friend on La Palma and will attempt to get my robust mountain papayas through the winter, partly outside and partly inside in the stairwell.

Papayas grow well in normal or garden soil. According to Chester D. French and my other books, they don't like too much water since the fleshy roots of the papaya begin to decay if they become too moist. For this reason, they recommend soil that is quite permeable to water and air. Another suggestion they make is adding ten to twenty percent sand to normal soil. However, Harald Tietze recommends not adding any sand: "Papayas like a lot of compost; flowerpots for small papaya plants only need to be about 8 inches deep, for large house plants (up to 8 feet tall) it would be ideal to have containers which were 24 inches deep, which one can place in a water basin with a water level of two to four inches, without damaging the plants." (Harald Tietze's letter to me dated July 1, 1997).

I took his advice to heart, and since my "Babaco" and my mountain papaya have wet feet, they appear to be doing well: they don't have any more yellow leaves. But you should try this out for yourself. The papaya comes from a humid, hot climate. The cleaned or purchased seeds sprout best in special plant-rearing soil (which can be obtained from the garden center) at a soil temperature of 72 to 86 degrees Fahrenheit after three to four weeks. I have had a positive experience with a small room greenhouse that I can slide open during the day and close at night. A windowsill without direct sunlight has proved to be an ideal location for it. The plants should be watered with soft water or rainwater at room temperature.

If you use a room greenhouse, the plants must be hardened for about two weeks before they are planted outside. Every day, open the ventilation flaps at the top of the greenhouse a bit more or slowly remove the greenhouse lid so that the seedlings can adjust to the unaccustomed dry air. I didn't do this the first time I planted papayas. Because of the beautiful summer weather, the plants literally dried up because they couldn't close their pores, which were wide open and suited to the previously humid air, quickly enough.

Even if you live in a cooler climate, you can still put your papaya tub plant in a warm, sunny, wind-protected area outside (such as on the south side of a house) during the summer.

Papaya plants are usually either male or female, so you need at least two of them to obtain fruit. The flowers can be pollinated with a brush. If the plants are outside, the wind and insects will do this work for you. The bisexual plants can form the fruit on their own.

The plants can be fertilized every week during the growth phase with a 0.2 percent solution of organic liquid fertilizer or, when they are planted outside, with compost or organic fertilizer. They need to be watered on a regular basis.

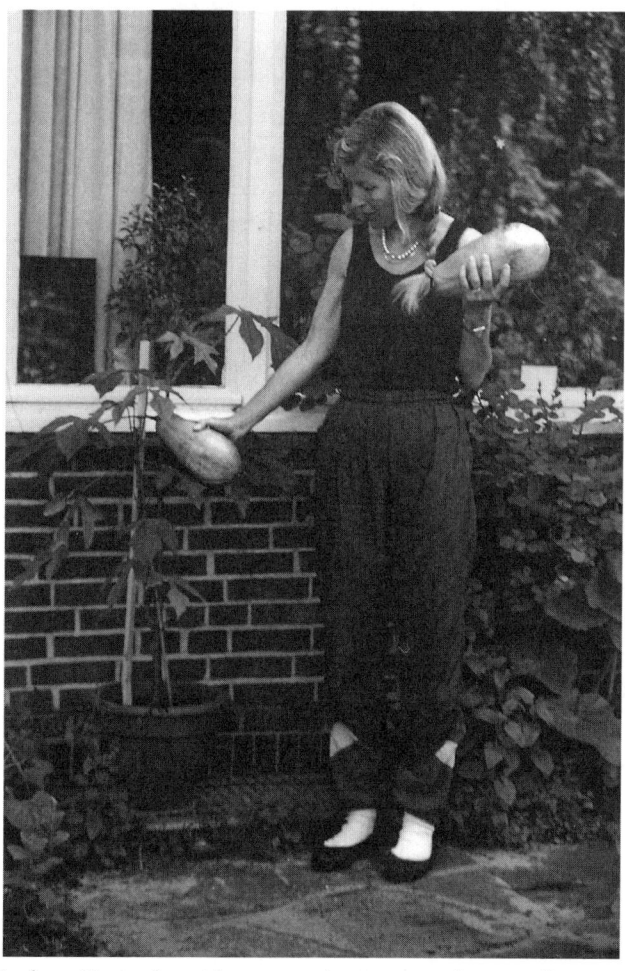

Barbara Simonsohn with a mountain papaya and papaya fruit in Hamburg, Germany

What's in the Papaya?

"A papaya a day keeps the doctor away"
("The Maui News" from November 23, 1992)

The Cubans call the papaya *fruta de bomba*. This fruit really is a knockout when it comes to its vital ingredients—the vitamins, minerals, trace elements, and enzymes! Not even all of the enzymes and other active components have been researched. Many authors think there are thousands of enzymes, biocatalysts, that have not yet been discovered. The most complete list of the papaya's contents is found in the essay "The Chemistry and Biochemistry of Papaya" by Professor Chung-Shih Tang, the papaya specialist at the University of Honolulu (see *Bibliography*). In view of the great diversity of application possibilities for the papaya, Tang believes there is a "knowledge gap in the therapeutic value of the papaya plant" and that there must be many other biological components in addition to papain that are therapeutically effective. As an example, he mentions carpaine and pseudocarpaine, two alkaloids present in all green parts of the plant and its seeds. These have been studied for a long time as a heart medication and, more recently, as a cancer medication (also see *Cancer—Causes and Alternatives* on page 95).

All orange-colored, yellow and red exotic fruits contain a large amount of beta-carotene, vitamin C, flavones and roughage materials such as pectin, volatile oils, and amaroids and tannins, which cleanse our "insides" of pollutants and also kill germs. This is why these fruits have made it to the top of the hit list in US cancer information brochures. They activate our metabolic processes, as well as stimulate the nerves, brain, and mind. They also have a proven antidepressive effect. The papaya's abundance of provitamin A protects against cancer and heart diseases, in addition to strengthening the immune system.

Among the exotic fruits—grapefruit, papaya, tangerine, avocado, orange, kiwi, banana and lemon—papaya has the most carotenoids: 3.44 mg per 100 grams of edible fruit. The main carotenoids are lycopene and B-cruptoxanthine. Papayas with red flesh contain only half of the carotenoids found in the pulp of the yellow fruit.

Ingeborg Muenzing-Rulf—German author of a book on healthy nutrition—praises the papaya in particular. This fruit should be eaten at breakfast because "it stimulates digestion and is rich in provitamin A, vitamin C, potassium, calcium and other regulative substances."[29] The nutritional values for the papaya vary with different authors. Here is a nutritional analysis from the book of Dr. Michael T. Murray, a representative of Natural Hygiene (also see *Bibliography*):

Contents of a Papaya	approx.	500 grams
Vitamins:		
Provitamin A	approx.	2.80 mg
Vitamin C	approx.	420.00 mg
Vitamin B1 (thiamin)	approx.	0.15 mg
Vitamin B2 (riboflavin)	approx.	0.20 mg
Vitamin B3 (niacin)	approx.	1.75 mg
Vitamin B6	approx.	3.50 mg
Vitamin H (botin)	approx.	0.10 mg
Minerals:		
Potassium	approx.	1300.00 mg
Calcium	approx.	120.0 mg
Iron	approx.	2.0 mg
Magnesium	approx.	200.0 mg
Phosphorus	approx.	80.0 mg
Sodium	approx.	14.0 mg
Protein	approx.	2.0 g
Carbohydrates	approx.	10.0 g
Fat	approx.	4.0 g

This means that the papaya is enormously rich in antioxidants such as carotene or provitamin A (more than in carrots), which protect the cell against free radicals—they contain more vitamin C than kiwis or carrots!—and flavonoids. Antioxidants protect us from cell degeneration and the related diseases such as cancer. Flavonoids regulate the permeability of the blood vessels. In addition, papaya contains many minerals, particularly potassium, magnesium, and calcium in natural, organic form. It has been established that the calcium from fruit and vegetables can be utilized much better by the body than calcium in inorganic forms or milk products. Consequently, papayas can be particularly recommended to women for preventing osteoporosis. The selenium content varies between 0.8 and 2.8 mg per 100 grams of edible fruit.

The overall sugar content of the ripe fruit is between 32 and 45 grams per pound of fresh weight. Half of this is saccharose, about 30 percent is glucose, and about 20 percent is fructose. The acid content of papaya is very low, so it can be used even when the stomach is irritated.

The mountain papaya, which is native to Columbia and Ecuador, thrives at heights of 7,900 to 9,200 feet above sea level. It has a relatively low sugar content: 0.99 percent glucose, 0.33 percent fructose, and 1.01 percent saccharose. Yet, its aroma is unique, pleasant, and intensive.

Because of the large amount of literature available on this topic, I would like to present only a brief summary of the most important contents of the papaya:

Most important contents of the papaya

Name, Properties Known Effects ....
.... *Symptoms of Deficiency*

Vitamin C—Water-soluble, strengthens the immune system and connective tissue, kills bacteria responsible for tooth decay, as cancer prevention, relieves pain of lumbago, strengthens muscles ......
.... *Bleeding gums, scurvy, colds, overweight, loss of hair, lack of concentration, sleep disorders, varicose veins, hemorrhoids, impaired vision, delayed healing of wounds, weak heart, depressions, bruises*

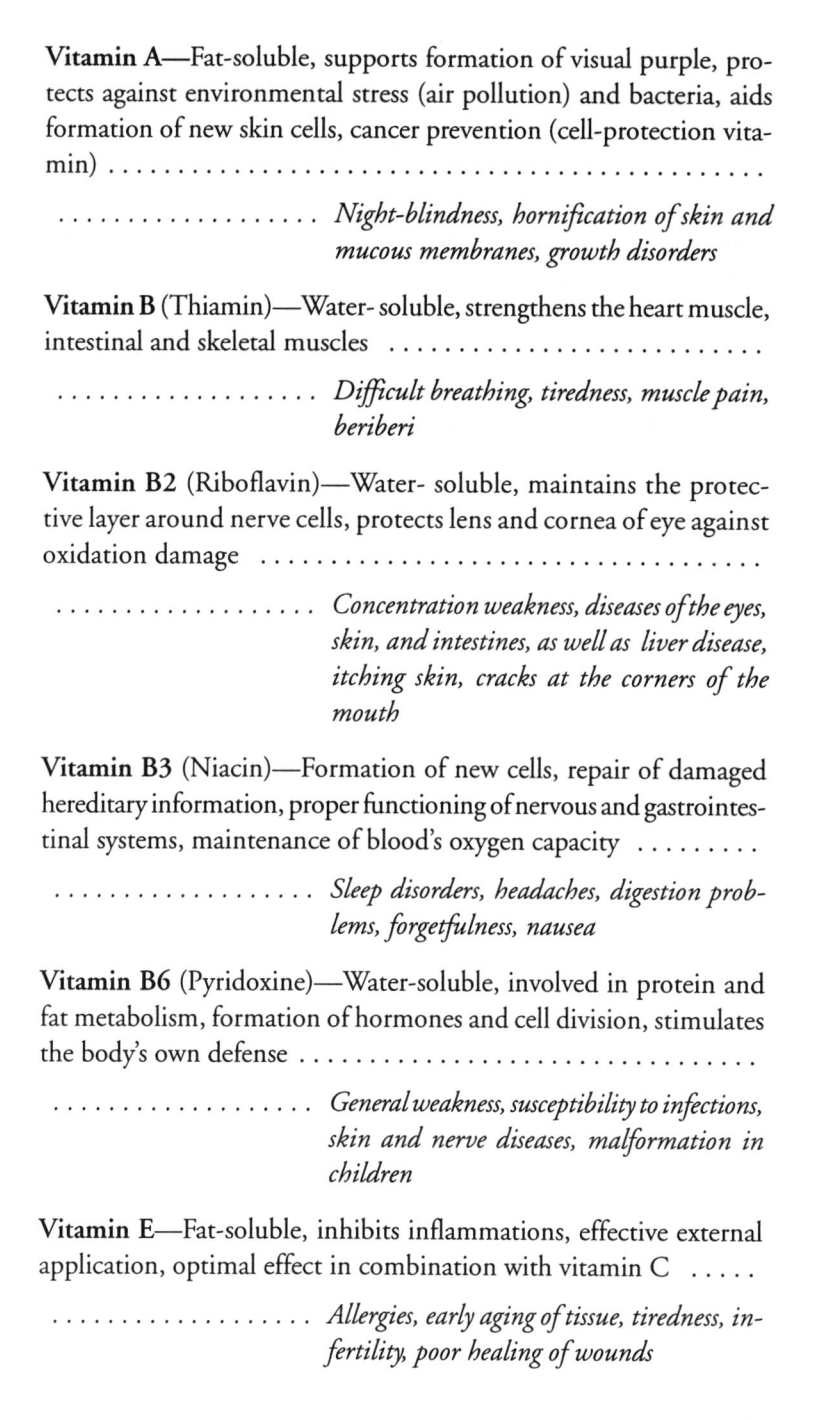

Vitamin A—Fat-soluble, supports formation of visual purple, protects against environmental stress (air pollution) and bacteria, aids formation of new skin cells, cancer prevention (cell-protection vitamin) ....

Night-blindness, hornification of skin and mucous membranes, growth disorders

Vitamin B (Thiamin)—Water-soluble, strengthens the heart muscle, intestinal and skeletal muscles ....

Difficult breathing, tiredness, muscle pain, beriberi

Vitamin B2 (Riboflavin)—Water-soluble, maintains the protective layer around nerve cells, protects lens and cornea of eye against oxidation damage ....

Concentration weakness, diseases of the eyes, skin, and intestines, as well as liver disease, itching skin, cracks at the corners of the mouth

Vitamin B3 (Niacin)—Formation of new cells, repair of damaged hereditary information, proper functioning of nervous and gastrointestinal systems, maintenance of blood's oxygen capacity ....

Sleep disorders, headaches, digestion problems, forgetfulness, nausea

Vitamin B6 (Pyridoxine)—Water-soluble, involved in protein and fat metabolism, formation of hormones and cell division, stimulates the body's own defense ....

General weakness, susceptibility to infections, skin and nerve diseases, malformation in children

Vitamin E—Fat-soluble, inhibits inflammations, effective external application, optimal effect in combination with vitamin C .....

Allergies, early aging of tissue, tiredness, infertility, poor healing of wounds

Potassium—Vitally important for proper heart function, protein and carbohydrate metabolism, activation of various enzymes ....

Weakness of heart muscle, loss of appetite, constipation, nausea, difficult breathing

Calcium—Important for bones and teeth, blood coagulation, stimulation of nerves and muscles ....

Osteoporosis, broken bones, rachitis, cramps, weak kidneys

Magnesium—Construction of bones and teeth, function of nerves and muscles, lowers blood lipid concentration ....

Muscle twitching, cramps, vomiting, heart palpitations, feeling of numbness

Phosphorus—Regulates acid-alkali equilibrium, important for teeth and bones ....

Muscle weakness, bone problems, growth weakness

Sodium—Cell function, regulates water content and acid-alkali equilibrium ....

Lack of motivation, vomiting, lack of appetite, low blood pressure, muscle cramps

Iron—Important for oxygen supply of the blood ....

Anemia and depigmentation, tiredness, grooves in fingernails, split hair

Enzymes—
The Magic Potion for Joy,
Health, Beauty, and Youth

Life isn't possible without enzymes. Enzymes are active ingredients vitally necessary for plants, animals and human beings. All life processes are an ordered and integrated sequence of enzymatic reactions. Enzymes are called "biocatalysts," which means that they activate and facilitate life processes such as respiration, cell division, and digestion. In these processes, each enzyme has a very special task and may become active up to 36 million times within one minute. Every process that is "activated" by an enzyme in the body occurs on an average of one million times more frequently than processes without them.

The word enzyme comes from the Greek: *Zumé*—which means "yeast." In 1897, Eduard Buschner discovered the first enzyme in beer yeast; he called it "Zymase" and later received the Nobel Prize for this discovery. Since then, about 4,000 enzymes have been studied more closely. However, scientists assume that there are about 40,000 enzymes involved in all life processes on earth.

Every unheated plant or animal food is full of the enzymes required for complete digestion, such as those for breaking down plant fibers. These enzymes are destroyed when cooked, inhibiting the digestion of fat and protein. By eating denatured "fast foods," preserved foods, and instant meals, we subject ourselves to the danger of using up our own body enzyme reserves too early.

Dr. Edward Howell has noted the importance of a sufficient enzyme supply. He believes that each of us is given a limited supply of bodily enzyme energy when we are born. He compares this energy supply to that of a new battery, since it must last a lifetime: The more quickly we use up our enzyme supply, the shorter our lives will be. He points out that much of our enzyme energy is wasted haphazardly throughout our lives since the habit of cooking our food and eating it processed with chemicals—as well as the use of alcohol, drugs, and junk food—all draw upon huge amounts of enzymes from our limited supply.[30]

If you nourish yourself without enzymes, you force your body to steal from its reserves in order to maintain enough pancreatic fluid and digestive juices. This results in a shortening of life, diseases, and reduced resistance to stress. When raw foods are eaten, the body's reserves remain available for combating illness. Dr. Edward Howell points out that among all the creatures on our planet, only human beings and their pets nourish themselves so that they are deficient in enzymes, vitamins, and minerals.[31]

Wild animals are not overweight; they do not suffer from cancer and rarely from other diseases. He designates the human race as "half sick". To spare the pancreas, which secretes the pancreatic fluid rich in enzymes, he particularly recommends raw fruits and vegetables: In order to obtain enough enzymes from our nutrition, we must eat food without heating it since heating food to more than 122 degrees Fahrenheit destroys valuable enzymes. Our largely enzyme-free food also no longer contains even the "building blocks" from which the body could produce its own enzymes.

Vitamins, minerals, and trace elements serve as so-called coenzymes, or enzyme helpers. Our absorption of an adequate amount of coenzymes is also endangered by the depletion of the soil and our modern nutrition with its abundant low- nutrient fast-food but too few raw foods. Consequently, there is not only a widespread lack of magnesium and selenium, but also of iron and Vitamin C. Smoking, medications, alcohol, environmental toxins, and continuous stress rob our bodies of their vital substances and choke off the activity of enzymes.

As we get older, the body's own enzyme production is reduced: for example, that of the pancreas is reduced by about 60 percent. This means that digestive disorders develop and the immune system is weakened. At the age of 40 at the latest, most people suffer from enzyme deficiency.

Enzymes in the Papaya

The unripe papaya contains many more types of enzymes than the ripe fruit: the protein-digesting enzyme papain, chymopapain, and papayalysozym. The thin-skinned papaya needs these enzymes while it ripens to repel insects. "Without these killer enzymes, the papaya would not be able to survive the subtropical jungle battle."[32] The papaya does not keep pests out with a hard skin like the pineapple, but fights using chemical weapons from the inside. Papaya enzymes are "natural drugs" and fully harmless.

Gene researchers have recognized the central value of our protein metabolism: Every process that influences our physical and mental or emotional health takes place through protein. Vitamins, fatty acids, trace elements, and all the other nutritious components serve only as aids in protein metabolism. However, for many people it is precisely this vital metabolic process that is disturbed: they lack sufficient hydrochloric acid, and the pancreas of almost everyone older than 35 years of age no longer produces protein-splitting enzymes at full speed. Stress, inadequate exercise, and above all, an improper diet with too much animal fat, sweets, and too little fruit and vegetables are the causes of this enzyme deficiency.

Enzymes are heat-sensitive and destroyed by boiling, baking, and frying. This means that we use up the body's enzyme supply too early, resulting in poor protein utilization and other problems: Undigested protein decays in the intestines, the intestinal flora deteriorates, intestinal toxins get into the blood, cells and glands are no longer supplied with the necessary nutrition, and our immunological system is weakened (also see *Intestinal Health* on page 87 and *Papaya as a Digestive Aid* on page 91).

Dr. Geesing talks about an "immune pause" after the 35th year of life: We should rebuild our supply of enzymes at this time in order to arm ourselves against infections and avoid becoming the victim of chronic illnesses.

The authors Klaus Oberbeil and Dr. Christiane Lentz list the following effects of papaya under the heading of "Healing with Papaya":
• Improvement of the protein status in all body cells
• Vitalization, strengthening, and restoration

- Reversal of protein-insufficiency disorders
- Activation of muscle formation, strengthening of heart and circulation
- Activation of hormones, more libido and joy
- Strengthening of immune system and mucous membranes

Doctors advise "papaya treatments" for this reason. The cells are revitalized by the papaya like a piece of parched land that has longed for rain. You can already feel this invigoration after just a few days: You need less sleep, feel mentally more alert, and generally in a better mood and more fit—even early in the morning!

Professor Chung-Shih Tang from the University of Honolulu, Hawaii, has determined that the broad application spectrum of the papaya in folk medicine allows us to conclude that, in addition to the enzymes, further bioactive components exist in the plant. There is an enormous lack of knowledge regarding the active chemical components of the papaya.

Enzyme Therapy

According to the Bible, a fig paste was used more than two thousand years ago as a healing remedy. Even at that time, people were aware of the healing power of enzymes, in this case that of the ficins of figs. "And Isaiah said: Bring a plaster of figs! And they brought it and laid it on the gland; and he was healed." (II Kings, Chapter 20:7). According to Ebstein (1901), the fig plaster also played a role in Germany in its simple form: "The fig is softened in milk and applied to inflamed areas of the mucous membrane of the mouth."[33]

According to Hoppfe (1975), the green fruit of the fig tree *(Ficus Carica L.)*, which is related to the *Carica papaya*, contains a pungent-tasting milky juice with albumin, mineral salts, the ferment cradin, enzymes, and an alkaloid-like compound that inhibit the growth of sarcomas (tumors of the connective and supportive tissue). In other tropical fruits there are also protein-splitting enzymes, the so-called protease: actinide is in the kiwi, bromelain in the pineapple, and the even more effective enzyme papain, as well as chymopapain and caricain (the latter has not yet been used for medicinal purposes in Europe), are in the papaya.

In raw papain, the enzyme proportions are: 30 grams of chymopapain, 5 grams of papain, 26 grams of caricain, and 28 grams of glycylendopeptidase. Fresh pineapple, kiwi, and papaya help in weight reduction because they stimulate the metabolism, force the elimination of waste from the body, and break down protein more quickly. Both metabolism and digestion function better as a result. The Indians of Central America, who ate pieces of papaya after heavy meals in order to aid digestion, already knew this (also see *The Discovery and Propagation of the Papaya* on page 32 and *The Papaya in the Ethno-Medicine of Native Peoples* on page 132),

Enzyme Preparations

In 1900, the first medical experiments to heal with enzymes took place in the West. In the beginning, plant and animal enzymes were injected and, until the middle of the Twentieth Century, research was restricted to hereditary enzyme defects and occasionally cancer tumors as well (also see *Papain in Enzyme Therapy against Cancer* on page 103). Since the beginning of the Sixties, enzyme preparations have been available for self-medication in health food stores and drugstores, usually without prescription. Enzyme preparations have no side effects, and an overdose isn't possible since excess enzymes are excreted with the bowel movement.

The Federal Drug Administration (FDA) rated Systematic Enzyme Therapy as GRAS (= generally recognized as safe). Its safety was rated similar to that of food.

When you buy enzyme preparations, be sure that they have a protective coat that cannot be destroyed by hydrochloric acid. Then the intestine can take full advantage of their full effectiveness.

There are enzyme preparations available at natural food, health food stores, and pharmacies that contain only papaya enzymes, as well as mixtures of plant enzymes. Plant enzymes are primarily used to eliminate digestive disorders. There are also preparations containing only papain that are safe worm remedies, even for children. In addition, papain and bromelain reduce swelling, help heal injuries and chronic inflammations, and degrade pathological immune complexes (conglomerates of antigens and antibodies) in autoimmune diseases. They are capable of breaking down these enormous protein molecules and eliminating them.

In addition to papain and bromelain from pineapple, many enzyme preparations also contain enzymes of animal origin such as pancreatin, trypsin, and chymotrypsin. Animal enzymes can break apart solid blood clots and remove the individual fragments via the blood.

In combination, these mixed enzyme preparations cover many areas of application and exhibit no side effects at high dosages when taken over longer periods of time. Systematic enzyme therapy naturally activates the self-healing powers of the body and strengthens the immune system. Consequently, many doctors recommend combined enzyme preparations as prevention to strengthen the defense system, to replenish the enzyme supply, and as a preventive measure when there is danger of sport injuries or before an operation. As a course of treatment, enzyme preparations should be taken twice a year for one month at a time.

The application areas for **Systematic Enzyme Therapy** are:
- Aging problems
- Arthritis
- Burns
- Cancer
- Capillary diseases such as varicose veins and arteriosclerosis
- Danger of miscarriage (after consulting gynecologist)
- Dental operations (also as a preventive remedy)
- Digestive disorders
- Embolism
- Gastric and intestinal ulcers
- Herpes
- Infarctions
- Infections
- Injury (for athletes and as a preventive remedy for sports)
- Intervertebral disk deficiency
- Mastopathy (breast problems)

- Multiple Sclerosis (MS)
- Operations (take 1-3 days beforehand as preventive remedy)
- Ovarian infections
- Rheumatism
- Thrombosis

Many additional syndromes and the latest research results can be found in books written by Howell and by Chichoke on systematic enzyme therapy.

Enzymes intensify the effect of antibiotics when taken together. If you want to combine them, consult your healthcare practitioner or doctor, particularly if complaints develop. When hiking or traveling, I always take along an enzyme preparation and an enzyme-containing ointment to be better armed for possible injuries to my children or myself and accelerate the healing process. The enzyme ointment disinfects, and I have successfully applied it to my daughter's dry skin areas and skin changes related to food allergies. It is also said to work well against herpes and skin inflammations.

Enzymes have the big advantage of not suppressing the immune system like many rheumatism and cancer medications (the so-called immune suppressives) but strengthening our resistance. They dissolve pathological immune complexes, eliminate dead cells and water accumulation more quickly, and improve the supply of nutritive substances to the cells. In addition, pain is relieved: the pain is not suppressed, but its cause is dissolved. Success with systematic enzyme therapy against cancer and AIDS patients gives hope (also see *Papain in Enzyme Therapy against Cancer* on page 103). Enzymes can increase the amount of time between infection and the outbreak of AIDS, reduce the symptoms, and improve the quality of life for the afflicted person. In cancer patients, reduction of side effects from orthodox medical treatment, strengthening of the lowered resistance, prevention of the feared formation of metastases, and activation of a cancer-destroying defense molecule, tumor necrosis factor TNF has been observed.

Dr. Max Wolf, author of the book *Enzyme Therapy* and founder of systematic enzyme therapy points out that because of a lack of enzymes the body is aging earlier.[34] On the basis of our genetic program, we should be able to become at least 120 years old, yet we only manage an average of 80 years for women and 78 for men. Particularly when we get older, we should eat a lot of raw foods, rich in enzymes and coenzymes, get enough exercise (see *Sport is Suicide?—Movement is Life!*, on page 20 and be sure to maintain a balanced, stable psyche (also see *Emotional Health: Stress, Get Lost!* on page 24).

Life can only come from life. It makes no sense to eat denatured, overcooked food and then take a few enzyme pills to balance things out. The legendary longevity of peoples who still live in harmony with nature—like the Hunzas—is primarily attributed to the high portion of enzyme-rich raw foods. In the words of Helmut Wandmaker: "We need unaltered natural food with its magnetic, electrical, living effect that bears its spark plug, the enzyme, within itself! This is the entire law of nature for human beings and animals!"[35]

There is currently an "enzyme wave," offering a great number of enzyme preparations in pharmacies and health food stores. Preparations containing the enzymes of tropical fruits such as the papaya and pineapple are also enjoying great popularity as weight-loss remedies.

It's a good idea to take enzymes after a cooked and especially after a heavy meal. However, it would be even better to reduce the consumption of cooked food and meat and cheese and eat more enzyme-rich raw foods. For people who have a weak digestive system (including many older people), enzymes are a great help. But we should guard against becoming "pill-takers." Helmut Wandmaker points out the clear and drastic psychological dangers of consuming enzyme medication: "You take pills so that you can 'deceive' yourself. Many 'experts' from the nutritional sector, as well as some physicians, recommend these preparations! They know that their patient is 'guilty,' but they also know a way around this self-betrayal." And doesn't a fresh papaya or pineapple or a salad with sprouts taste ten times better than tablets from the bottle?

Papaya Juice: A Health Cocktail

"The strength of your body lies in the juice of plants."
(Shin-Nong, Chinese emperor, author of the world's oldest book on healing plants, about 3700 B.C.)

Nutritionists and doctors recommend that we eat more fresh fruit, salad, and vegetables in general. Making juice is one of the simplest methods for reaching this goal. Juices have the big advantage of providing easily digestible plant nutrition in a concentrated form. Fresh fruit juices and vegetable juices supply us with valuable vitamins, pure water, enzymes, minerals, trace elements and additional, still undiscovered active components. Less than ten percent of Americans and Europeans follow the advice of experts to eat at least two portions of fruit and three portions of vegetables per day. More than forty percent do not eat fruit or drink juice, and almost half don't eat garden vegetables every day. In view of the six million cancer deaths per year and the probable doubling in the number of cancer patients during the next 25 years, the World Health Organization called for a change to a new, healthier lifestyle in its 1997 report. Even by the year 2005, it is expected that the number of lung cancer cases will increase by one-third for women and prostate cancer cases will increase by 40 percent for men in the European Union.

It has been determined that people who consume at least sixty percent of fresh plant foods in the form of fruit, seeds, vegetables, and fresh juice, live longer and are more likely to be free of degenerative diseases. Juices are digested within minutes. In contrast to the tired and "dead" feeling after eating cooked or fried food, we feel fresh, healthy, vital, and dynamic after eating!

When we do not include fresh juices, it is difficult to obtain the food we need as prevention against cancer, heart diseases, diabetes, and infarction. As an example, for cancer prevention the recommendation is as much provitamin A or carotene as would be obtained from two-and-a-half pounds of carrots or papayas. This is the equivalent of about six large carrots or two-and-a-half papayas. Wouldn't it be easier to drink one-half liter of carrot or papaya juice? Perhaps fresh juices are an alternative to the expensive nutritional supplements that are increasingly offered.

Dr. Norman W. Walker lived to be 116 years old. To the very end, he was physically and mentally active and had no diseases of old age. In his book *Raw Vegetable Juices*, he notes that freshly squeezed juices are not a concentrated food. Juices are fluid foods that contain top-quality pure, organic water without requiring dehydration. Their water concentration has not been reduced.[36] Juices are full of vitamins and enzymes. Since the human body rapidly absorbs them, they are astonishingly quick at renewing the entire organism.

Juicing simplifies the digestion process. It allows us to absorb food more rapidly, even within minutes. The result is that we quickly have more energy! Consequently, juices are especially suited for patients, small children, and older people. They also greatly benefit people with damage to their digestive organs that normally prevents them from eating raw foods. In addition, we can fast with juices to remove waste materials, cleanse the intestine, and regenerate the detoxification organ.

To fast with juice, drink only fresh fruit juices and vegetable juices, preferably from organically cultivated products. Papaya particularly stimulates elimination, removes waste materials, and cleanses the intestines. Apart from freshly squeezed juices, drink just water. Then you will have a greater sense of well-being and feel charged with energy. Many tips for juice fasting can be found in the book *How to Keep Slim, Healthy, and Young with Juice Fasting* by Dr. Paavo Airola.

Here are some of the benefits of fasting with juice (recommended by Dr. Hermann Gerhard and Dr. Juergen Weilhofen in their German-language book on the topic):

- Removal of waste materials and cleansing of blood
- Intestinal cleansing and balancing
- Stimulation of eliminatory organs like the liver and kidney
- Relief for heart and circulatory system.
- Activation of the self-healing powers
- Reduction of excess weight
- More self-confidence and beauty

- Decrease of risk factors such as high blood pressure, high blood sugar, and high cholesterol values
- Preventive health care
- Rejuvenation of body cells
- Prevention of early aging
- Revitalization
- Expanding the horizon of experience.

"Zero-food" fasting causes hyperacidity as a result of ketones flooding the body (resulting from the degradation of fats). If you have had negative experiences with this, you will probably have no problems with juice fasting. The carbohydrates in the juice break down the ketone bodies even further so that no metabolic "traps" develop. We have more energy available to us during juice fasting because fresh fruits and vegetables have abundant vitamins, minerals, and trace elements.

It isn't easy to obtain organically cultivated tropical fruits in all areas. Perhaps this book will help increase the demand for unsprayed papayas so that more organic farms can be organized in subtropical areas! Some dealers have specialized in exotic, organically cultivated fruits, which are comparatively expensive. According to information from several dealers, papayas generally have less artificial fertilizer applied to them and they are not sprayed as much as other tropical fruits such as bananas.

Walker recommends the robust and long-lasting "Champion Juicer" as an ideal juicer. It grates and presses at the same time so that all the active ingredients are optimally retained. He claims that this device extracts vitamins, minerals, and other active ingredients from fruits and vegetables, retaining the enzymes more completely than any other method. The "little brother" of the "Champion Juicer", the "Suco," is somewhat less expensive and small enough to easily take along when traveling. I have also found the Champion Juicer to be very reliable. For example, it's quite easy to use and clean. A mixer isn't suitable for extracting juice since it also mixes in all the fibers, which are difficult to digest and often full of residues.

Above all, fruit juices and vegetable juices contain water-soluble fibrous material. This lowers the cholesterol level. Bottled juices only fulfill a small portion of the health requirements placed on them. Freshly squeezed juices contain enzymes that are lost in the pasteurization process. A large part of the vitamins and minerals, as well as other active ingredients that have not yet been completely researched, are lost in the preservation process. It has been determined that freshly squeezed apple juice contains enzymes with properties that are antiviral and inhibit viral reproduction; however, the apple juice sold at the grocery store does not have these properties.

Walter Schoenberger, founder of "fresh-plant therapy" as a system of healing, notes in his German-language book on juices that the fresh plant represents a uniquely harmonious "specialty," a biological unity. This unity has a much more positive effect than dried drugs or chemical products. The juice from the fresh cells of the complete plant is not only capable of fighting the symptoms but also guides the function of the entire body in natural, and therefore healthy, directions. Investing in a good juicer is an investment in your health!

Juices can be stored for about 12 hours and taken in a thermos bottle as an energy drink to your office, for example. Children, who sometimes don't like fruits and vegetables, love freshly squeezed juice. They like to help make the juice. My son Michael, age 11, concocts his own "fantasy" drinks or healthy ice cream himself. Then he decorates the juices with colored straws, peppermint leaves or orange slices and pieces of pineapple. Instead of the sweetened unhealthy school milk, he drinks the juice that I fill into a small thermos bottle to keep it fresh. As a result, he feels fit, alert, and full of energy even at the end of a long school day or during strenuous tests. Walker explains that vitamin and mineral preparations usually contain only one active ingredient. An example of this is beta-carotene: Preparations containing beta-carotene are useful but only contain one type of carotene. Juices have contain a broad range of carotenes, many of which are stronger antioxidants and cancer inhibitors than beta carotene.[37]

Dr. Norman W. Walker and Jay Kordich in particular started a real "juice fever." Kordich is convinced that he can conquer cancer with a diet of 13 glasses of carrot-apple juice per day. After he was healed, he decided to inform people about the power of juice. He developed a reasonably priced juicer, the "Trillium Juiceman." Forty years later, Kordich is still convinced of the advantages of freshly squeezed juices.

Norman Walker reports a similar healing success by drinking raw juices. He also survived a severe illness with the help of fresh carrot juice, leaving him in better condition in his old age than when he was thirty. His doctor considered Walker's recovery in eight weeks to be "phenomenal". From that time on, Walker restricted himself to a healthy diet of raw salads, vegetables, and fruits, which he supplemented with large quantities of raw juice whenever possible. He particularly emphasizes the rejuvenating effect of a healthy diet. In terms of intestinal cleansing and regeneration of the entire glandular system, the papaya plays a key role for him. His definition of what it means to be young touched me deeply. "To be young means having all or most of the attributes of youth, health, energy, vitality, and perpetual laughter on the lips and in the eyes. It means being genial, cordial, curteous and polite to everybody, irrespective of creed, color or social status. It means being constantly active, with many irons in the fire if necessary, so that there shall never be one moment which weights heavily on one's hands. (...) To become younger we need Vitality. Vitality is not merely the temporary display of activity, of quick motion or of nervous outpourings. It comes from a deep-rooted sense of rest, poise, awareness and strength which makes one feel *on the top of the world* and that life is truly worth living every waking moment."[38]

Walker praises the very special therapeutic value of the papaya's juice. According to him, papain from the fruit has the same effect as the pepsin in our digestive process. Today it has been established that papain, which is particularly active in the still unripe papaya, supports the formation of fibrin. This in turn promotes the healing of wounds. Walker enthusiastically reported on an injury that could scarcely be seen the day after it was covered with a compress made of the pressed paste of a green papaya (including the skin). He was able to once again use his finger, which had been seriously squeezed by a machine, two days after the treatment. Walker claims that both the green and the ripe papaya juice are unbeatable for most physical disorders.

I naturally don't want to give the impression that papaya juice can heal everything. A healthy, balanced lifestyle, with good nutrition and exercise on a regular basis, is also important (see *Sport is Suicide?—Movement is Life!* on page 20) as well as a truly positive view of life. Walker has pointed out the negative effects of the "poison" adrenaline on our body functions. We can eat (or drink, author's addition) the best food in the world but this will not prevent the deterioration of our body if we are constantly caught up in anger, fear, cares, frustrations, and negative moods.[39]

In their books on juice, both Murray and Walker have A-to-Z sections with recommendations about what juice is most suitable for each problem. However, the authors make clear that treatment of disease belongs in the hands of a doctor or healing practitioner and juice cannot replace medications. If you only drink fresh juice and otherwise pay no attention to your diet, you will be unsuccessful. Juices have their—important—place within the scope of a comprehensive and holistic health program. They should also be given a recognized place in schools, kindergartens, hospitals, hotels, restaurants, and homes for the aged.

Effects of Papaya Juice on Our Endocrine and Exocrine Glands

Health and a ripe old age aren't possible without our glands functioning in a normal manner. Glands influence not only the release of hormones but also our emotional life. We learn from Dr. Norman Walker the following about the glands:

1. **Thymus gland**
   The thymus gland controls the carbon metabolism, corpus luteum and thyroid gland, parathyroid gland and adrenal gland, and menstruation. It stimulates the uterus. Functional disorders may result in excessive menstruation: the function of the sexual glands is then affected adversely. Walker recommends the juice of ripe papayas.

2. **Corpus luteum** (menstruation and pregnancy gland)
The hormones released by the corpus luteum control menstruation and pregnancy. Functional disorders may result in miscarriages and menstrual disturbances. Walker recommends the juice of ripe and green papayas.

3. **Ovaries**
The ovaries control menstrual functions, formation of egg cells, and milk secretion. They stimulate the adrenal glands, pineal gland, pituitary gland, thymus gland, and thyroid gland. Functional disorders may result in the formation of cysts and tumors. Walker recommends papaya juice.

4. **Liver**
The liver controls oxidation (accumulation of oxygen), oxygenation (transfer of oxygen), and elimination of toxins. It stimulates the lymph glands, pancreas, and spleen
Functional disorders may result in acidosis (hyperacidity), an increase in blood pressure, and an irritation of the peripheral nerve endings. A. Vogel, a well-known Swiss naturopathic physician, points out the papaya's healing power and good tolerance for liver patients repeatedly in his books. Walker recommends the juice of ripe and green papayas.

5. **Pineal Gland**
The pineal gland controls the development of the sexual hormones and the sexual organs, as well as intellectual and mental development. It stimulates the sexual organs. Functional disorders may result in hyposomia or gigantism. Walker recommends the juice of ripe papayas.

6. **Follicle**
(Egg sack: egg-cell bearing portion of ovary)
The follicles control femininity, hair growth, and optimistic moods. They stimulate the adrenal glands, the anterior pituitary lobe, the corpus luteum, the thymus gland, the nervous system, and the liver. Functional disorders may result in pessimism or mental imbalances. Walker recommends papaya juice.

7. **Lymph glands**
   The lymph glands control the sulfur metabolism. They stimulate the spleen. Functional disorders may result in the formation of pus and toxemia (excessive toxins). Walker recommends ripe papaya juice.

8. **Spleen**
   The spleen regulates the sulfur metabolism, filters wastes from the blood, and revitalizes cells and tissue. It stimulates the lymph glands. Functional disorders may result in high blood pressure and premature aging. Walker recommends papaya juice.

9. **Adrenal glands**
   The adrenal glands control the suprarenal cortex and therefore the anabolic calcium metabolism. They stimulate the mineral balance and influence the sugar content of the blood and the immune reaction. In addition, they regulate the sexual functions, menstruation, and the release of vitamin C. They stimulate the muscles, nervous system, and the process of building and regenerating cells. Functional disorders may result in cramps, intestinal disturbances (irritable colon), low blood pressure, and tumors. Walker recommends the juice of green and ripe papayas.

In conclusion, here is another thought by Walker on the topic of "gland care" through proper nutrition on all levels. He says that the physical, emotional, and mental care of the body is very important. If one of these levels is neglected, a catastrophe cannot be avoided. Our endocrine glands help us attain and maintain radiant health. See *Bibliography* on page 217, Dr. Norman Walker: *The Natural Way to Vibrant Health*.

Juice Recipes

Pure papaya juice tastes great. Here a few variations of mixtures from Michael T. Murray's book *The Complete Book of Juicing*. I have tried them out myself, but don't set any limit to your own imagination! By combining them with other fruits, you can benefit even more from the valuable ingredients of these fruits and enjoy a diversity of tastes.

1. **Papaya-Pear:** Remove seeds from half of a papaya, cut into slices, and add two sliced pears.

2. **Papaya-Pineapple:** Remove seeds from half of a papaya, cut into slices, and add half a sliced pineapple with skin.

3. **Apple-Papaya:** Cut two apples into pieces and add half of a sliced papaya (without seeds).

4. **Orange-Papaya:** Peel two oranges and add half a sliced papaya (without seeds). This looks great if you use blood oranges. Try serving the juice in a champagne glass with a straw, a slice of orange, and a few a lemon balm leaves.

5. **Grapefruit- Papaya:** Peel a grapefruit and cut half a papaya (without seeds) in slices.

6. **Potassium Punch** is a great way to begin the day with lots of vitamin C, B6, and potassium! Remove the core from a peach and cut into slices. This recipe also requires two peeled oranges, half a sliced papaya (with seeds removed), and a peeled banana. First juice from the peach, then one of the oranges, then the papaya, and finally the second orange. Pour the juice into a mixer, add the banana, and then liquefy the contents.

7. **Enzyme cocktail:** This super breakfast is a great way to begin the day and tastes delicious even without banana. It has lots of vitamin A, C, E, and thiamin (B1), as well as vitamin B6 and potassium! Remove the core from half a mango. Peel two oranges. Cut a papaya in half, remove seeds, and cut in slices. Cut half a pineapple in pieces with peel. Remove skin from a banana. First juice the mango, then one orange, the papaya, the second orange, and finally the pineapple. Blend the juice with the banana until everything is liquefied.

8. **Ape Shake:** This is another excellent breakfast. Although low on calories (contains only 226 kcal), it is satisfying and can be appreciated by anyone with a "sweet tooth." This shake contains a lot of vitamin A, C, B6 and potassium, in addition to further vitamins

and minerals. First juice half a papaya (with seeds and peel removed) and then one or two peeled oranges. Pour the juice into a mixer and add the peeled banana. Then pour the thick juice into a glass and garnish with (organic) orange peels. My tip: If you want it even sweeter, add a few dates or raisins to the banana.

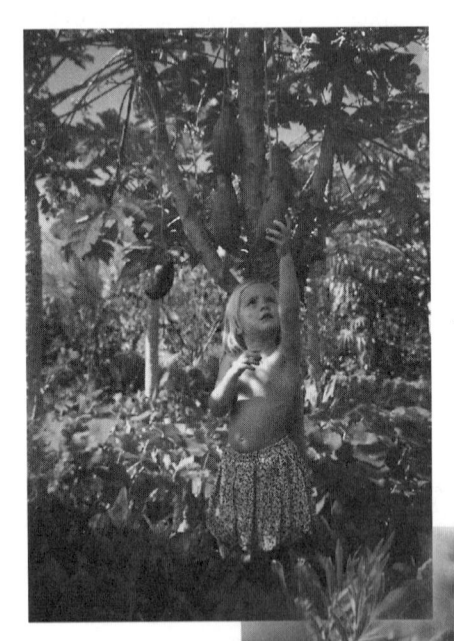

Freya, the author's 3-year-old daughter, beneath a male papaya tree on La Palma

Michael, the author's 9-year-old son with fruit on a female papaya tree

Papaya—A Fountain of Youth

"The papaya is the fruit of a long life."
(Old Chinese Saying)

"The papaya is the Tree of Eternal Youth."
(Vasco da Gama)

Among other things, papayas contain an abundance of carotene. "People whose cell walls are packed full of carotene remain younger much longer than people with scanty carotene concentrations in their cell tissue."[40] With the "invention" of carotene, the plant world successfully developed the perfect defensive weapon against destructive free radicals. This makes it possible for plants to protect themselves against sunburn, hostile microorganisms, and aggressive substances like fungi, parasites, bacteria, viruses, etc. When we eat papayas and other orange-colored fruits and vegetables such as apricots, mangoes, pumpkin, and carrots, we protect our cells from oxidative damage. This could lead to premature aging, cancer, heart disease, cataracts, and clouding of consciousness.

Metabolic experts such as Dr. S. A. Mahmud have discovered that the Hunzas in Pakistan have astonishing longevity because they eat so many apricots. This fruit has revitalizing powers and strengthens the liver, qualities also found in the papaya.

Papayas and other fruits and vegetables containing carotene make us not only younger and healthier, but also more beautiful. This makes them an absolute must for anyone conscious of personal beauty. So put orange-colored and dark-green vegetables, salad, and fruits on your table every day! One to two papayas would be ideal.

Papaya helps you digest protein more quickly and thoroughly. At the same time, the body cells receive an abundance of valuable protein through the blood. "People live longer today, not because we have become healthier, but because we die more slowly."[41] We are biologically programmed for 120 to 140 years. But a diet rich in enzymes is a prerequisite for a healthy old age in any case. Our enzyme supplies need to be refilled. Fewer enzymes are produced when we are older, and they are of inferior quality. Enzyme-rich tropical fruits such as the papaya and other foods rich in enzymes like sprouts, algae, wild herbs, green juices, and garlic are recommended for this purpose.

If you aren't certain that your diet contains the necessary enzymes, you can include more raw food in your diet or you can do a preventive treatment (for example, with the enzyme tablets that can be obtained without a prescription from a pharmacy) on a regular basis for six to eight weeks twice a year. If necessary, you can take these remedies on a continuous basis without any harmful effects. This will lead to a general improvement in your health and productivity.

The papaya is believed to have a rejuvenating effect. Dr. B. Lytton Benard, who runs a health center in Guadalajara (Mexico), says that the cleansing effect of papayas isn't limited to the digestive tract. It reaches all the other tissue as well: "The key to rejuvenation and a long life in full possession of our powers lies in the papaya." Dr. Norman W. Walker also wrote that the papaya exerts a rejuvenating influence on all of our organs by harmonizing and stimulating our glands (see *Papaya Juice: A Health Cocktail* on page 59).

Halima Neumann presumes that the body protein arginine, which is influenced in its formation by papain, is responsible for the pineal gland's increased release of Human Growth Hormone (HGH). This hormone is important for cell-renewal processes and the regeneration of muscles, skin, cartilage, and liver. Walker also discusses the value of arginine: It helps to control the degeneration of body cells and protects the tissue against the formation of ulcers and cancer.[42]

To extend your life span, take the advice of Anthony Cichoke (author of *Enzymes and Enzyme Therapy*):
- Take enzymes and antioxidants such as vitamin A, E, C and selenium
- Eat a natural, well-balanced diet and eat mainly raw
- Get more physical exercise
- Maintain your normal weight
- Avoid drugs and environmental toxins

Papaya—Great for Sex!

I first came across the fact that the papaya stimulates almost all of the glands, including the sexual glands, in the works of Walker, my favorite author. (There is a summary of the effects on our glands at the end of *Papaya Juice: A Health Cocktail* on page 59). In a book by German author Klaus Oberbeil, I also found an allusion to the fact that papaya is good for the libido. Patrick Geryl lavishly praises the papaya and other exotic fruits in his book on sun foods, claiming that if you eat a lot of exotic fruit, you take in an abundance of natural aphrodisiacs and soon will overflow with romantic feelings. It's exciting to know that exotic fruits can lead you to a new life—to sparkling nights, a pounding heart, romantic affairs, and alluring adventures.[43]

Fruit Makes You Potent is the heading of an article by the British Advertising Bureau for Fruit and Vegetables. It goes on to comment that fruit has an extraordinarily positive effect on your love-and-sex life. Geryl discovered the effect of fruit on the libido years ago when he altered his diet to one primarily consisting of fruits. He says that if you have eaten fruit only occasionally up to now, it can help you get to know the erotic side of your partner. As a fruit-eater, you can lead an exciting, uncommonly satisfying sexual life, full of romance and the orgasms that you've always dreamed about. Their frequency, duration, and intensity will drive you nearly insane, he claims.

Dr. Abraham writes about his transition to natural sun foods and the consequences: "You feel 10 to 20 years younger, lose a ton of weight, and enjoy sex like you haven't experienced for years."[44] This effect of fruit can be easily explained: Enzyme-rich fruits give us an abundance of vital energy, which makes us more capable and potent. A living, energy-rich fruit diet even increases sperm production. "Even more astonishing is the fact that fifty-year-old men, who were completely or almost impotent, to their great surprise were able to enjoy an almost youthful potency."[45]

Geryl attributes the fact that fresh fruit can make tired old, tired people young again to increased hormone secretion by the sexual glands. It is reported that the Abchasians in Russia (a few of whom have lived more than 125 years), normally remain sexually active to an age of about 100 years. It is said that the Hunzas become parents at 60. The same also applies to the inhabitants of Vilcambambe, a mountain valley in Ecuador where the inhabitants reach an extremely old age. All of these peoples are vegetarians and a large portion of their diet consists of fruits and raw vegetables.

Dr. Edwin Flatto, author of the book *Super Potency at Any Age*, recommends a change to living foods for increasing the libido. He states that all cooked and canned food is dead. Dead food is everything that no longer has any life force. It no longer contains any oxygen, enzymes, or bioelectricity—in short, it lacks the essence of life.[46] Geryl says that such "sun foods" make women more active sexually. He attributes this to the enormous power of vitamin C and beta carotene.[47] The papaya contains an extraordinary amount of both these vital components (also see *What's in the Papaya?* on page 46).

Both nutrients revitalize the menstrual cycle so much that women who eat sun foods almost have no bleeding. (I have also had the same experience.) Menstrual problems belong to the past and new power is released in the form of "romantic energy." The plant hormones also help women cope with menopause. Both women and men eat at least two pounds of fruit per day—preferably bananas, papayas, mangoes, durians, peaches, and apricots. The hormones in the plants protect men from enlargement of the prostate and help them remain—or become—vital, potent, and full of life.

Beta carotene, whose chemical structure is similar to opium, stimulates sexual desire. Mangos, oranges, apricots, and tangerines are recommended in addition to papayas. Geryl writes that beta carotene converts blood cholesterol into sexual hormones with the support of the B vitamins.[48] B vitamins are also found in the papaya, and they are also abundant in strawberries, raspberries, and maypops. Geryl says it should be no surprise that we feel so well after enjoying an exotic fruit salad.[49] He is very enthusiastic about the "natural aphrodisiacs in fresh, exotic fruit juices" and writes that we can, as in a dream, feel one sensation after the other—sensations that we may not have thought possible until now.

Under the influence of exotic substances, the sexual center of our brain flips out and sends us back to our original state of wildness, just like earthquakes and volcanic eruptions shake entire continents. This ecstasy, triggered by the vitamins and minerals released by exotic fruits, will arouse us into erotic ecstasy.[50]

I hope that I haven't unnerved you with these quotations! I've even omitted the "hottest" sections. To reassure you: Scientists have proved that people who remain sexually active in old age are generally healthier and happier than their abstinent counterparts and usually outlive them. Sexual hormones stimulate our immune system, make us more beautiful, and defend us against stress, illness, and tension. With the help of the papaya and other tropical fruit, I invite you to activate your libido and to maintain a fulfilled sexual life into ripe old age. Through exotic fruit cocktails, you can improve not only your sexual potency but also your physical capabilities and desire to do sports. In turn, this will have a favorable effect on your love life.

What Ethnologists Discovered about the Erotic Aspect of the Papaya

An expert on China and Indochina told me some interesting things about the external use of the papaya as an aphrodisiac in this part of the world. I don't want to keep this information from the (adult!) readers of this book.

China

If you look closely at the Chinese characters for "man" and "woman," you will notice that they are simplified symbols for the masculine sexual organs—in the excited state—and the female sexual organs.

For thousands of years, the relationship to sexuality in China and Southeast Asia has remained astonishingly (and refreshingly) lighthearted and open in comparison to the West. For example, not only are the Chinese familiar with an "organ clock," indicating the times when the internal organs and glands are particularly active, but also an "erotic clock" with the different hours when males and females should become more sexually active. For women, this time is in the morning; for men it is in the evening. Special positions are used in relation to the day of the week. For example, one position is called "the Kaiser opens the jade lock"; another position is "the Kaiser greets the rising sun"—the vagina is reddened beforehand with papaya and henna; and a third is poetically called "the Kaiser enjoys the harmony of the butterfly."

Here is a fantastic notion for Western women: In the mountain tribes of China, the Meo woman expected to have at least three orgasms before the man approaches her with his own intentions. In order to extend this process, the vagina and the tip of the penis are rubbed with papaya sauce or papaya juice. The result is said to be a wave of multiple orgasms.

In China, dried pieces of papaya are still offered for sale in a small wooden box today. Some of these can occasionally be admired in museums of erotica. The boxes are painted with unmistakable motifs, and the two halves part like vaginal lips to show the contents when they are opened. Dried papaya pieces are placed into the vagina in the evening in order to stimulate erotic dreams. It is said that when the man rubs his penis with the juice of a ripe papaya his erection will last longer and react very sensitively to a tender touch. Supposedly, the woman will become aroused much more quickly with the help of the papaya.

A curious practice: In China, extramarital children have been extremely undesired for centuries because of inheritance reasons. The idea of women engaging in intercourse outside of marriage is therefore scorned. Even today, there are special sex salons where a lonely and unsatisfied woman can go anonymously—she enters and leaves through her own separate door. A pearl curtain hides the head of the woman from the curious eyes of the tea-drinking public while she experiences sexual satisfaction at the hands of a "master of the tongue." In addition, he smears papaya onto the vagina and clitoris, creating intensive stimulation so that a series of orgasms flow into one another. The woman pays nothing for this experience, but those present (six to eight) men—sometimes even a woman watches—must pay an entrance fee equivalent to $4.00. They are also entertained by the master's erotic stories. You find stimulating information on how to enrich your sex life with the help of papaya in Linda Jaivin's bestseller "Eat Me!", released by The Text Publishing Company, Melbourne and Broadway Books, N.Y., 1995.

Chinese character for "woman"

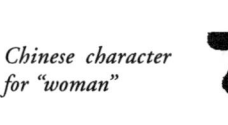

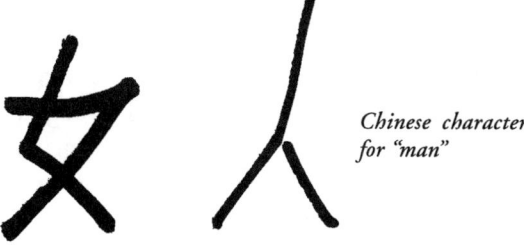

Chinese character for "man"

Indochina

A doctor, who worked in a hospital in the province of Quang-Nam near Hue during the Vietnam War, told me the following experience. A woman from the tribe of Rhades was brought in one evening with injuries caused by a mine explosion. In the process of taking care of the hip wound, he observed a clear secretion and a piece of papaya slid out of the vagina. The vulva appeared to be highly aroused. A Vietnamese nurse commented that the woman was apparently on the way to her lover and had inserted the papaya as an erotic means of shortening foreplay before the actual act of intercourse.

A Spanish doctor told me that men and women in Spain sometimes also use the papaya for sexual stimulation. We can assume that the papaya enzyme stimulates the hormonal nervous system.

Central America

In 1996, a friend of mine was responsible for a ship's pharmacy and the medical care of its passengers and crew during a sea cruise in Central America. He successfully treated a patient who had a vaginal infection with watery discharge resulting from multiple acts of sexual intercourse within a short time by applying a papaya cream from Honduras.

This ointment has an extensive spectrum of applications ranging from scurvy to vaginal infections, rectal problems like hemorrhoids, and general mucous membrane infections. The Indians of Central and South America have known the antiseptic effect of the papaya for several centuries (see *The Papaya in Ethno-Medicine of Native Peoples* on page 132 and *Papaya against Inflammation* on page 115).

In Puerto Rico, my friend treated an older woman successfully with a papaya ointment, which was available in drugstores and herb stores for the equivalent of $2.00. The woman had an uterus prolapse, in which the uterus is pressed through the vagina because of overexertion of the ligaments. This problem is normally operated on. After four-and-a-half days, the woman had no further difficulty with it and could continue her trip.

Thailand

A young acquaintance of mine went on an "erotic vacation" to Thailand in 1996. At a massage salon specializing in certain erotic practices, he had himself pampered by three women, one after the other. Thanks to a papaya ointment (which he nicknamed "smear soap" because of its green color) that the two women from Thailand and a woman from China rubbed on their vaginas, as well on his penis, he had no problem achieving an erection after two orgasms. He even had a third "dry" climax. In this situation, the "antibiotic" and conception-preventing effect of the papaya certainly played a role for the otherwise completely unprotected women. However, until papaya has been proved to be 100% effective against HIV, people should continue using the customary safe-sex practices!

I received this information "at the last minute" before completing the book, so that I haven't tried out the papaya as an external aphrodisiac yet myself. I certainly won't prevent readers from experimenting on their own with this topic.

Help against Acidosis (Hyperacidity)

"Hyperacidity of the body is the basis of all diseases."

(Paracelsus)

In a nutrition book for pregnant women that he wrote in 1913, the Norwegian biochemist Ragnar Berg recommended that we should normally eat four times as many alkali-forming as acid-forming foods; when we are sick, we should eat seven times as much of alkali-forming foods. Modern eating habits take exactly the opposite approach: the civilized diet consists primarily of acid-former foods like bread, meat, milk products, white flour, cola soft drinks, sugar, coffee, and alcohol. Only 20 percent consists of alkali-formers such as fruit, vegetables, potatoes, herb teas, and mineral water. No wonder that most people in Western industrial nations are "hyperacidic."

A large variety of studies have shown that 90 percent (!) of the population is much too acidic, leading to an abundance of negative health factors.[51] Stress, too little sleep, and inadequate physical activity all lead to acidosis. In earlier ages, people engaged in hard physical labor that caused them to exhale or sweat out the acids. An acidic body environment also leads us to easily react harshly, get mad about trivial things, be overcritical, and express little love or joy in life. Even in the early afternoon, we feel exhausted, impatient, and unambitious—up to the point of the "burn-out" syndrome. This is because a healthy mind can only exist in a healthy body.

The hyperacidity of the organism also extends to the emotional state. When this acidic condition is corrected through a deacidification treatment, a person's mood may brighten so much that even severe depressions disappear. Today, an acid-alkali equilibrium exists almost exclusively in babies and in people who live in countries entering a period of famine.

We all tend toward "latent acidosis." Latent acidosis or creeping hyperacidity, in which the tissue gradually accumulates acids, is the basis of civilization's diseases. This makes itself evident, for example, in slight mucous-membrane, skin, and periosteum allergies. Other symptoms may be dizziness, bad breath, an unpleasant taste in the mouth, a gray coating on the tongue or dark rings under the eyes. As a result of hyperacidity, free radicals are formed, destroying cell structure. Vitamins, minerals, and vital substances from foods are not utilized correctly and there are symptoms of deficiencies. The essential bacteria in the small intestine die, so that the immune system is weakened. Colds and all sorts of infections increase, as well as headaches and migraines. The hair loses its luster, there is an increasing tendency toward allergies (also see *Allergies* on page 111) and the skin becomes pale and sallow.

A healthy and normal metabolism can only occur within an alkaline environment. If a cell becomes too acidic, it dies. In his book about stored protein diseases, German author Lothar Wendt writes that animal protein—with the exception of raw milk consumed directly after milking—is metabolized as acid, causing the "acid death" of cells and living things in general. Enzymes, which are essential as biocatalysts for our metabolism, can only be effective when the cell environment has the proper acid-alkali relationship. The blood usually has a pH value of 7.4. Values below 7.0 and above 7.8 endanger life. With an increase in acidity, the blood can become so thick that it ceases flowing. This leads to a heart attack or cerebral stroke. At a blood pH value of less than 7.35, meaning an excess of acid, the condition is called "latent acidosis" or hyperacidity.

We can even avoid cancer through a markedly alkaline diet. Today we know that every person has cancer cells. But when these remain inactive, the disease does not appear. Cancer requires acidic surroundings for growth and existence. It cannot develop in an alkaline environment—just like carp cannot live in the sea and the shark cannot live in a fresh-water lake.[52] It's actually a scandal that hospital patients are served denatured, acid-forming food—even in children's hospitals and cancer clinics. I recently visited the Altona Children's Hospital and the Cancer Department of the General Hospital of Altona, Germany: The sick children and adults were given fruit only when they expressly asked for it! Salad was almost never served, not to mention organically grown fruit and vegetables. With this kind of diet, "only cancer and other illnesses of the patient's are fed—what terrible nonsense!"[53]

The pH value of a healthy person's morning urine lies between 6.0 and 7.4. Some pharmacies have inexpensive strips for measuring the acid content of urine—you can do this on your own! The lower the pH value, the more acidic the urine. (An extensive urine analysis to determine the acidity quotient, possible metabolic disturbances, and disorders of the kidneys and liver is done by some medical laboratories.)

The value of the acid-alkali balance depends on our food. This explains why there is no medication that can make us healthy when we don't feel well, are tired, and in a bad mood—the beginning symptoms of hyperacidity. Correct nutrition plays a key role as causal health care and is the basic therapy for every type of illness. An alkaline-based diet is the best protection against chronic illnesses and cancer.

When we suffer from hyperacidity, we become tired too easily. Doctors speak of neurodystonia (a disturbance of the nervous system) or a general state of exhaustion. Instead of resting and sleeping, many people take stimulants like coffee, black tea, cola soft drinks, or sweets, which in turn increase the acidic content of the blood. Ultimately, the afflicted person is forced by illness to rest and eliminate excess acids though the skin, the mucous membranes, the intestines, the bladder, and the kidneys. From this perspective, illness helps us to regain our acid-alkali equilibrium. Therefore, it is actually inadvisable to remove the illness signal "pain" with medication. With the exception of injuries, pain is primarily an expression of too much acidity in the body.

Cancer patients experience the greatest pain when the pH value in the vicinity of the tumor falls to 6.2. All of the cancer patients and diabetics I spoke to about the dangers of acidosis found their urine to be acidic when testing it. If we fight against pain instead of treating the cause, we behave like the driver who unscrews the oil-lamp indicator bulb so that he will not be irritated by it.

When the capacity of the eliminatory organs is exhausted, the body stores excess acids in the connective tissue and accumulates waste materials. The connective tissue forms the environment, the medium from which the cells nourish themselves. Among other things, its collagen fibers serve as an "acidic buffer" or "acidic reservoir." This prevents the dangerous acidic inundation of the body. Within this context, Glaesel speaks of a virtual primordial-kidney system of the mesenchymal connective tissue (the multipotent mother tissue of all forms of supportive and connective tissue).[54] The connective-tissue metabolism is damaged or blocked in all chronic diseases such as rheumatism, cancer, arteriosclerosis, and joint inflammations. The mesenchymal connective tissue should not be constantly stressed because it plays the key role in the metabolism and nutrition of all our organs, as well as immune defense. By pressing lightly on the outer side of the upper arm or neck, acidosis therapists and advisers can determine the extent of the excess acid accumulation and release the acids by applying a special connective tissue massage. When hyperacidity continues for a longer period of time, the body removes minerals from places like the bones and teeth in order to neutralize this acid. Perhaps this is one reason why osteoporosis (bone atrophy) has increased dramatically not only in older women, but also in children and teenagers.

A second reason lies in the loss of collagen fibers in the bones. The body stores excess acids not only in the connective tissue but also in the bones; this makes the bones more porous and brittle. In this regard, it is remarkable that in the countries where the most acid-forming milk products are consumed, such as the USA and Europe, osteoporosis is a major problem. In places like China and Japan, where almost no milk products are consumed, osteoporosis seldom occurs. Only raw milk that hasn't been pasteurized or homogenized is alkaline for a short time. Next to wheat, milk is the most common food allergen (see also *Allergies* on page 111). For children, the increasing consumption of soft drinks plays a role in the loss of calcium from the bones and hyperacidity of the blood.

Nutritionists like Dr. Paul Bragg and Dr. Paavo Airola (see *Bibliography* on page 213) believe that acidosis as the main cause of all types of diseases. The regulation of the acids and alkalines has a life-sustained function for us. A regulated metabolism depends on acid-alkali equilibrium. When the normal process of physiological exchange is too greatly disturbed, a person becomes sick.

We can see a similar development in trees damaged by acid rain: At first glance they still appear to be healthy ("apparent health"). But when we examine them more closely, we see the thinning of their crowns, which is a sign of illness and the death of healthy cells. Trees weakened by acid rain are susceptible to other diseases such as fungi and lose their ability to regenerate (also see *Papaya Combats Fungal Disease* on page 116).

The intestine is the root of the human plant. Just as soil is important for trees, our food is the most important environmental factor for our bodies. Similar to the situation of the trees, the dangerous thing about "nutritional sins" is that the connection between nutrition and health is often not recognized: errors in nutrition only become apparent in the form of health disorders after years or decades.

We eliminate excess carbon dioxide through our lungs when we exhale. (It is transported to the lungs via the blood in the form of bicarbonate and in a globulin complex.) The excess acids in food are a burden to the kidneys and eventually lead to poor concentration and metabolic disorders. These are the main reason for epidemic outbreaks of chronic diseases, the cause of which are considered to be virtually unknown. For this reason, they must practically be viewed as non-healable. Therapies in which people place much hope, and therefore become fashionable, have their limitations if they do not simultaneously reinstate equilibrium in the mineral metabolism and acid-alkali balance.[55]

Diabetes is also a typical "acid disease" in which the metabolism of carbohydrates and fatty acids becomes disrupted. As a result, ketones are formed, leading to acidosis. Fats are not completely digested, creating acidic compounds. Diabetes is the most widely spread disease leading to acidosis.[56] In the later stage of their illness, diabetics are often "acidic" psychologically as well. The acid-alkali equilibrium plays an important role in all health disorders because it influences the blood pressure, capillary circulation, and all of the other metabolic processes. Consequently, the enzymes necessary for life only function as biocatalysts within a narrow pH region. Most illnesses also begin with failure of the enzymatic mechanism. This initially leads to a functional disorder before morphological, pathological changes occur.

Green and ripe papayas, together with their seeds, can greatly aid in reestablishing and maintaining the acid-alkali equilibrium. As early as 1945, the American researchers Dr. John Kellog and professor Lafayette B. Mendell of Yale University discovered that papaya with its enzyme papain is a top-ranking natural remedy in terms of its alkali-forming effect. Digestant pills containing papain not only help in more easily digesting proteins, fat, and starches—they also reestablish and maintain the acid-alkali equilibrium. However, we might as well eat either the green papaya or the ripe fruit! Both the ripe and the unripe papaya are strongly alkali forming, as well as very healing for the liver and stomach. Moreover, the entire unripe papaya and the seeds of the ripe papaya contain the strongly alkalizing compound carpaine in addition to papain.

Even people who do not tolerate acidic fruits because of fruit acids and are forced to avoid them can eat papaya and organic bananas. These individuals have problems with uric acid and often suffer from gout or rheumatism. With the help of the very alkaline papaya, they can quickly break down the internal acid deposits and reduce their symptoms. It's also important to follow the rules of food separation (see *Fit for Life* by Harvey and Marilyn Diamond). Carbohydrates and proteins should not be eaten at the same meal in order to avoid decomposition and fermentation processes in the stomach ad intestines that can lead to further hyperacidity.

The special and positive feature of green and ripe papayas is that they can be eaten together with either proteins or carbohydrates! In Halima Neumann's German-language book on acidosis, there is a table showing what foods can be combined. In the table of "Alkaline and Acidic Effects of Foods," green and yellow papayas have by far the most alkaline effect of all fruits on our metabolism! The positive value is around 20. As a comparison, a few values are listed for other fruits: apple 3, banana 5, strawberries 2, oranges 6, and grapes 3-6. The alkaline effect of the papaya is only attained by algae and spirulina (20-25), as well as dandelion leaves, dried figs, and currants (20). The only foods that form more alkalis are cucumbers (30) and fresh olives (35). Since papayas taste very good and sweet, we can generally eat larger quantities of them than these other foods.

For the information of those interested in nutrition, I would like to list the most intensive "acid-forming" foods: fish (-20), meat (-20 to -25), meat extract (-50), baker's yeast (-50), cheese spread (-20), kefir cheese (-17), roasted nuts (-10 to -20), white rice (-18), and wheat flour (-15). Alcohol, coca soft drinks, coffee, and black tea are also strong acid-forming foods and should consequently be only consumed in limited amounts as well. Green tea, herb teas, and non-carbonated mineral water are alkaline.

On the subject of enzymes, Halima Neumann wrote: "The million-dollar business with protein-splitting enzyme tablets—usually with papain, bromelain, and pancreas extract from animals—doesn't eliminate either the body waste or the deposition diseases, but is only a cover-up method."[57] Therefore, eating papayas or pills made from papayas shouldn't be viewed as an alternative to a healthy life style and proper nutrition. However, it can help us to increase and support the reorientation of our body in the direction of the acid-alkali equilibrium in order to aid the healing process and remove its (acidic) basis.

In the long run, we should do without strong acid builders such as meat products since these are digested in the intestine by putrefying bacteria, which release poisons resulting from decomposition. Consumption of milk products should also be limited because of their acidic effect—Lothar Wendt speaks in this regard of the danger of "protein-deposit diseases" and Bruker cites the "protein bomb" in kefir (curd) cheese.

One very important way of countering hyperacidity is relaxation, which simultaneously reduces stress and therefore breaks down acids. I enjoy using Authentic Reiki, a simple and very effective method of deep relaxation. After just one hour of Reiki treatment, I have discovered a considerably reduced degree of acidity in both my own urine and that of others. When our blood is in an alkaline state, we can think more clearly, enjoy making decisions, and are mentally alert. An acidic condition inhibits the activity of the nervous system, while an alkaline condition stimulates it. The following changes will be noticed by anyone who conquers hyperacidity with alkaline-based proper nutrition, relaxation methods, and stress reducers (like autogenic training, meditation, and Authentic Reiki, the Radiance Technique), activity in the fresh air, visits to the sauna, resting periods, and, if necessary, an acidosis therapy with connective-tissue massages and intestinal cleansing according to Dr. Collier:

- Less health disorders
- Reduction of pain
- Decrease in inflammatory processes
- Sleep disorders disappear
- Increase in powers of concentration
- Reduction in susceptibility to infection, colds occur less frequently
- Decrease in tiredness and exhaustion, replaced by more initiative, cheerfulness, vitality, and joy in life
- Deep spiritual experiences.

Personal Experiences

When I was in my mid-20s, I was exhausted and had no drive. I felt like an old woman. Everything was too much for me. I couldn't afford this in terms of my work either since I was a public relations manager. I thought I was properly nourished with whole foods. Back then, I didn't know that even whole foods with a large proportion of milk and grain products have an acidic effect.

At this time, I enthusiastically listened to Dr. Renate Collier hold a lecture on acidosis at the University of Hamburg during the "Alternative Health Days". Consequently, I registered for a four-week course of treatment at the sanitarium she ran on the island of Sylt at that time. As a result of the acidosis therapy developed by Dr. Collier— a system of connective-tissue massage, packs, bitter salts, and fasting with herb teas and mineral water (alternative: an alkaline diet), I literally became a "new person."

By the end of this treatment, I was so full of energy that I helped to massage Dr. Collier's "worst cases" without becoming tired and went bicycling by wind strength 6. Moreover, I experienced a mental alertness and clarity I had never known. My intestines were clean and healthy again, and my tissue was smooth and youthful.

Full of enthusiasm, I organized seminars with Dr. Collier, did treatments on a regular basis, and increasingly monitored my acid-alkali equilibrium. I trained to hold acidosis seminars and become an acidosis consultant so that I could pass on knowledge about the origin and treatment of this health disorder.

Here are the most important tips:

- In many tropical and subtropical countries, people usually eat half a papaya at breakfast. This is a good idea since the body is usually slightly "acidic" mornings after the nighttime cleansing.
- All freshly squeezed fruit juices and vegetable juices are alkali forming. Particularly in the morning, you can enrich them with the very nutritious spirulina algae powder or wheat-grass juice, which is also strongly alkaline. People with a wheat allergy can use barley (also available as a powder), but it is much richer in vital substances if you make it yourself in a juicer.
- If you have meals containing animal protein, you should eat ripe or green papayas with them. An alternative is using the digestive aids made from the papaya, usually available in health food stores.
- The proportion of raw plant foods should basically be increased in the diet, which means five (small) meals a day containing fruit and vegetables. In this way, we automatically attain the acid-alkali equilibrium and prevent diseases caused by civilization such as heart attacks and cancer.
- We should allow ourselves a raw-food day as often as possible so that the body remains slightly alkaline: eat only raw, uncooked food and give preference to alkaline foods like papaya and carrots or make algae drinks from chlorella, blue-green, or spirulina algae, "the green manna". All wild herbs and sprouts are also very alkaline. A juice day has a similar effect.
- The Japanese Shinto religion recommends taking a cold bath or a cold shower in a river, waterfall or the sea. If you take warm showers, you should always use cold water at the end in order to alkalinize the blood and other body fluids. Hot showers and baths make the blood acidic, but cold water makes it alkaline. Cold showers make me very active and improve my brain functioning. In addition, they strengthen the will power and the ability to make decisions, as well as improving the mood. They help with stress and problems. It can take ten days before these positive effects become noticeable. Hold out, it's worth it! I now only take cold showers in the morning and feel refreshed and in a good mood for hours.

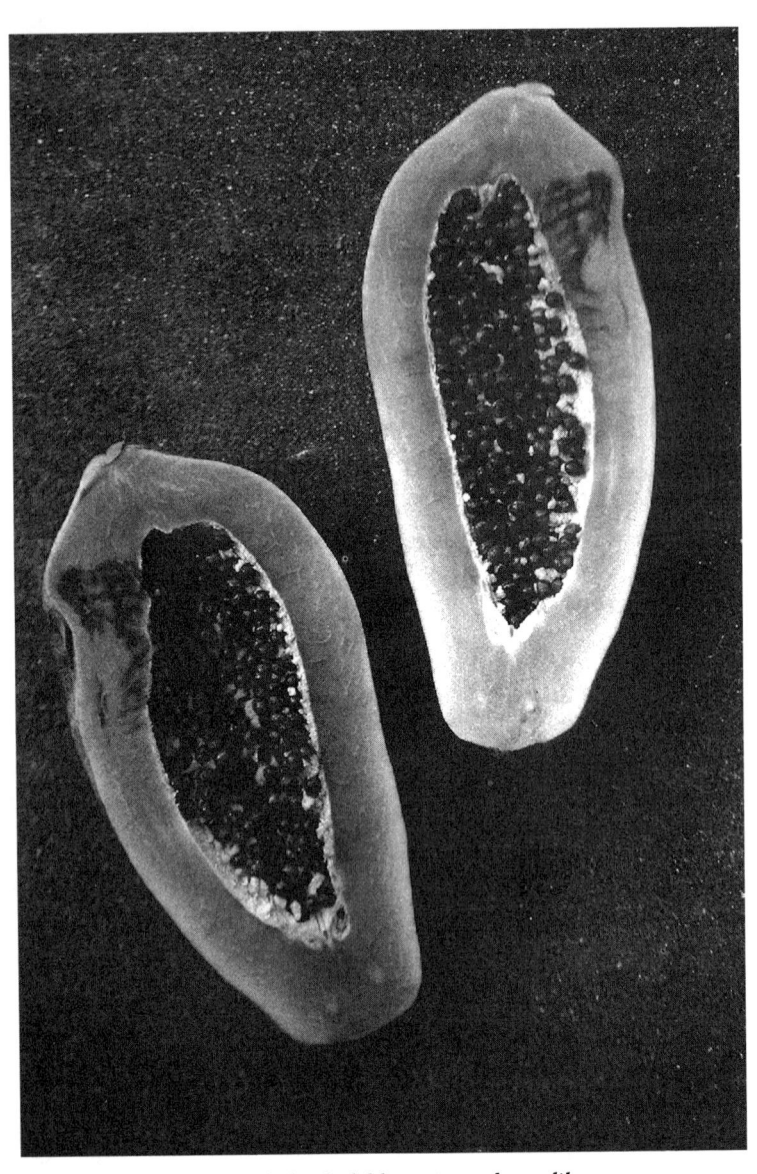

Ripe papaya with dark seeds that look like caviar and taste like cress.

Intestinal Health

"The intestine is the root of the human plant"
(Franz Xaver Mayr)

*"The intestinal juice reflects the food;
The blood reflects the intestinal juice;
The flesh reflects the blood."*
(Boerhaave, 1740)

Our digestive system begins in the mouth and ends with the anus: It is a 6.5 meter long system with a total surface area of 300 square meters, as large as a tennis court and therefore our largest area of contact with the outer world! In our digestive system, our food is taken apart with the help of intestinal bacteria, absorbed, and metabolized in order to provide our cells with vital energy. This intestinal flora is very important: in experiments, animals raised in a germ-free environment survived only for a maximum of 90 days due to the missing intestinal flora.

Healthy intestinal flora is also invaluable for our immune system and provides protection against bacterial infection. Professor Nissle observed during the First World War that soldiers who had a particular strain of Escheria coli bacteria in their large intestine were protected against dysentery and other intestinal infections. Vitamin K, biotin, and the B vitamins can only be absorbed when there is a population of certain coli bacteria. An imbalance of bacteria in which pathogenic (illness-causing) germs gain the upper hand is considered to be the most common cause of immune weakness. We should therefore always strive to have healthy, efficient intestinal flora. This means the optimal symbiosis of the bacteria necessary for life in a disturbance-free, metabolically active milieu for the mutual benefit.[58]

Nutritionists and physicians have long agreed that uncooked food such as fruits, nuts, grains, and vegetables are the healthiest diet because they reduce the quantity of toxic substances produced in the intestine.[59] Cooking destroys every type of enzyme, which is present in fresh foods and an excellent digestive aid. Consequently, a "mixed diet" leads to illness and causes imbalance, degenerating and disrupting the natural intestinal flora.

When we eat large quantities of animal protein, putrefaction processes occur in the intestines. Meat is decomposed by putrefying bacteria and remains in the intestine for up to 90 hours. Toxins, poisonous substances, wander through the intestinal wall into the body. In the process of decomposing animal protein, ptomaines, which are some of the strongest poisons, are formed, as well as ammonia. The latter poisons the brain metabolism and leads to a chronic decrease in vitality. Instead of blood being supplied with high-quality nutrients for the cells, it accumulates fermentation poisons. All fermentation processes leave behind waste products, which form deposits on the intestine walls. These years of layers become hard and impermeable. We "starve in front of full pots."

Overeating also leads to digestive problems: "Enjoy being moderately full and blessings and reason will prevail." (Goethe) Tips for slow, meditative meals can be found in Omraam Mikhael Aivanhov's book, *Yoga of Nutrition*. The evening meal should not be too late because: "The intestine goes to sleep with the chickens and gets up with them" according to Franz Xaver Mayr, the famous German intestinal specialist. When we eat too late, we feel poisoned or drugged the next morning because the intestine begins to actively work in the morning: the decomposition poisons of the food that has lost its value through the overnight fermentation enter the blood stream. Consequently, Halima Neumann recommends only drinking fluid foods after 7pm. For example, make a spirulina drink (very tasty): one teaspoon of algae powder, one teaspoon of brewer's yeast, and a pinch of tamari stirred into a glass of lukewarm water.

There is a beautiful Arabian quotation about the amount of food that we should eat: "God has set aside for each at his birth a certain amount of food and drink; he who enjoys little at a time will live from it for a long time; he who requires much will soon have nothing left." The smallest common denominator of those who live to a hundred years is in most cases the moderate intake of food. My grandfather, who turned 104 in 1999, has only an indentation where others have a stomach and appears to be made of skin and bones. Yet, in spite of this, he is still able to work in the garden, including turning up the soil with a shovel!

You can check how long food requires to pass through your intestine when you eat food with pigments such as spinach, spirulina algae, or red beets and wait until your bowel movements show the corresponding color. Food should never remain in the body for longer than 12 hours. When the digestive process proceeds physiologically, no gas is formed and the stool has a light color (unless you eat spirulina algae!) and almost no odor. Chronic constipation or diarrhea indicates a sick intestine. Deposits on the intestinal walls can even let hair roots "starve" and lead to loss of hair or early graying.

The enzymes in papayas help to split and digest proteins quickly and without problems when they are eaten with meat and other protein meals. In his book on nutrition for fighting cancer, the German professor Dr. Leitzmann recommends serving a piece of papaya with meat dishes in order to digest them more easily. As a result, it is possible to avoid autointoxication, when the putrefaction poisons diffuse through the intestinal wall into the blood, and the papaya's protein-degrading enzymes can dissolve existing waste deposits in the intestine. Figs and pineapples also contain this type of protease, as well as raw sauerkraut, onions, garlic, and fresh herbs. On the other hand, salt is considered to be an "enzyme inhibitor." Cooking, as well as preparing food in the microwave, destroys enzymes.

German author Wolfgang Spiller considers intestinal autointoxication, the self-poisoning of the intestine, as the "most common principle that causes diseases."[60] Sebastian Kneipp, a 19th century German naturopath, commented that "all illness has its origin in disturbances of the blood, whether its circulation is disrupted or its composition is ruined." Only a healthy intestine guarantees health, well-being, a strong immune system, and a good metabolism. If you would like to allow your intestine to rest and want to free it extensively from putrefactive bacteria and waste deposits, you should fast and cleanse the intestine or have a colon-hydrotherapy treatment on a regular basis. If you eat one tablespoon of papaya seeds every day for four to six weeks before you plan to have colon hydrotherapy, the waste deposits in the intestinal villi will be softened and dissolved. This means that you will only require about half the number of these relatively expensive treatments.

Walker in particular points out how the condition of the intestine is related to stress and nervousness. He notes that it is almost impossible to keep a clear head and the correct emotional and mental equilibrium if we haven't taken care of our large intestine for a while.[61] There is a close relationship between the pituitary gland, which is our "master gland", and the appendix, along with other body functions. Walker has discovered that colonic irrigation could prevent many more physical and emotional disorders than most people realize. However, it is also important to drastically reduce the consumption of meat: Enzyme preparations and tropical fruits should not "misused" for continuing to engage in nutritional sins without suffering any health consequences.

In the long run, we can only become healthy and stay healthy when we eat a proper diet. Many people take better care of their cars than their bodies! No driver would ever think of filling the tank with lead-free super instead of diesel if that's what the car requires. The same driver is often proud of tolerating any kind of food and can't understand why his mental and physical capabilities are constantly diminishing and that he is increasingly plagued by minor complaints and, ultimately, chronic disease.

Here are some of the symbiotic foods that help develop healthy intestinal flora: all kinds of fruits and vegetables, including salads, all edible nuts and seeds, all types of grains and sprouts, vegetables pickled in lactic acid, sour-milk products (not suitable for those with allergies), springwater with low mineral content, tea (except for black tea), fruit juices, and vegetable juices. All foods should be chewed well so that they are completely soaked in saliva: Digestion begins in the mouth!

Here is the "blacklist" of foods and other substances hostile to symbiosis that should be restricted: sugar, refined flour, industrial fats, meat, fish, poultry, eggs, pasteurized and homogenized milk and milk products, industrially prepared baby food, sugar, preservatives, dyes, flavoring, artificial aromas, coffee, black tea, alcohol, and nicotine.

In summary, the following basic rules should be observed:
- The more natural and less processed the food is, the better it is for the digestive system.
- The more thoroughly food is chewed and soaked in saliva, the easier it is on our enzyme system and the better it will be metabolized.
- The fewer animal products you eat, the better.

When we take control of this symbiotic process by eating a healthy diet and cleansing and maintaining a healthy intestine this affects not only us, but also our children and their children. Our parents and grandparents not eating a proper diet probably have caused defects in our own immune system and contributed to our metabolic disorders. Allergy experts claim that the allergies from which 30 million people in Germany suffer are probably nothing other than "the last desperate cry for help from an organism battered for generations." Our children pay the penalty for our misguided behavior and that of our parents.

The books by Walker, Spiller, Ullrich, Neumann, and Glaesel (see *Bibliography*) document many case examples of people who radically changed their diets and utilized intestinal cleansing. As a result, they were even able to heal severe diseases and regain a long-lost vitality.

Papaya as a Digestive Aid

Professor R. H. Chittenden of Yale University was perhaps the first American scientist interested in the value of papaya for human nutrition during the 1930s. Many other researchers have since confirmed his observations.

A papaya enzyme breaks up the milk protein casein and lets it coagulate. In tests conducted by Dr. Frank Woodbury, it was proved that papain could liquefy such diverse foods as salmon, cookies, dry meat, halibut, potatoes, bread, peas, grilled sausages, cake, pudding, and cheese by adding papain.

In contrast to other enzymes, papain is effective as a digestant because it functions in both an acidic as well as in an alkaline environment. It is completely effective in both the hyperacidic stomach and intestine. The body can only use proteins when the stomach produces enough hydrochloric acid, which is also important for the absorption of calcium. The enzyme pepsin, which is often prescribed, can only aid digestion in an acidic stomach environment.

Once in the stomach and the intestine, the enzyme papain breaks open the meat fibers and speeds up the process of breaking down the proteins into amino acids, which the human body needs. The digestion of proteins includes many complicated chemical processes. As the various proteins are decomposed by the digestive system, the process goes through a number of intermediate steps until it is finally broken down by the enzymes into the actual basic building blocks of the cells, the amino acids. The amino acids pass through the intestinal wall into the blood stream, where they are initially carried to the liver. Only then can the organ cells begin with the synthesis of protein, the construction of valuable body protein that makes tissue formation and growth possible.

An inadequate biochemical processing of the protein substances leaves harmful decomposition products in the intestine. Many people have intestines teeming with putrefying bacteria that sustain themselves from the remains of simple protein bodies, usually of animal origin. Undigested protein remains can become so thick and hard that they impede the movement of the intestinal muscles—the intestinal peristaltic contractions. This can lead to self-poisoning—autointoxication—when deposits that have not been removed diffuse through the intestinal wall and enter the blood stream. They wander through the body and can cause complaints like tiredness, depression, and headaches.

This background information makes it easier to understand the significance of papaya and papaya preparations. Food waste deposits are thoroughly digested by the digestive ferment papain without painful flatulence and autointoxication. Putrefying bacteria are removed from the intestine; only in the presence of healthy intestinal flora can the essential vitamins and minerals—such as the "nerve vitamin" B12—be absorbed. Dr. Kellogg writes that papain is the only known fruit derivative that attacks and destroys dead cell tissue and repairs ailments such as ulcers.[62]

Halima Neumann recommends aloe vera leaves, either fresh or as juice, and freshly grated papaya herbage (possibly mixed with apple or a sugar-free applesauce), as a healing diet for people with stomach or intestinal ulcers.

Dr. David Chowry Muther, Mahatma Gandhi's personal physician, was convinced that infected stomach membranes (gastritis) and digestive problems could be quickly reduced through a diet containing papaya.[63] The elimination of hardened waste products from the large intestine also relieves the liver so that the heart is also indirectly alleviated. A swollen transverse colon often presses against the stomach and causes heart problems.

"When the organs gradually develop more difficulty in functioning at the onset of old age—or when a new organic weakness or injury occurs in addition to the occasional problems and these complaints mutually intensify each other—the papaya can help relieve and detoxify the entire organism in a particularly significant manner."[64] However, this measure should be accompanied by a change in the metabolic condition and avoidance of all previous nutritional errors. (This step also serves as a cancer preventive).

As an example of an important protein substance, arginine (one of the essential amino acids that the body cannot synthesize itself) can be obtained through papain from various kinds of foreign protein in the stomach and intestine. Arginine is present in very few foods, including eggs and brewer's yeast. It must be given to the body on a regular basis if the reproductive organs are to function properly. High levels of arginine inhibit the growth of cancer cells, particularly in the tissue of the breast and ovaries.

High blood pressure, constipation, flatulence, arthritis, and diabetes are examples of diseases and complaints aggravated by incomplete protein digestion. For this reason, papain-containing medications are used for such a variety of health disorders. These include stomach ulcers, gastritis, seasickness, children's digestion problems, skin diseases, nausea, worms, and some forms of anemia.

The story of the papaya and papain is similar to other great scientific secrets that have been discovered and lost again. In Jamaica, where papaya trees grow tall, the local population fed the fruit exclusively to chickens and pigs (in order to keep them healthy) but abstained from eating it themselves. They only started eating papayas after American scientists taught them about the value of the fruit, resulting in an improvement of their health.

Here a few tips:
- Remedies supporting digestion made from papayas are, for example, "Granozym" (natural food store), "Papayaforce" (Firm Bioforce), "Papayasanit-N" (Firm Weber & Weber) and "Papenz" (Vitaminera, USA). The last three medications are available from the pharmacy. In Australia Nature's Own "Papaya Enzyme" and "Charcoal & Papaya" (from Bullivant's Natural Health Products Pty. Ltd.) and Microgenics "Digestive Enzyme Formula" (from Optimum Healthcare Pty. Ltd.) are available in health food stores. See *Resources* on page 207.
- As an equivalent and inexpensive alternative, I recommend eating half-ripe papayas and the seeds of the ripe fruit (see *The Papaya as a Healing Remedy* on page 67).
- It's also possible to purchase a granulate from organically cultivated green papayas (for example, from Papaya John in Hawaii).

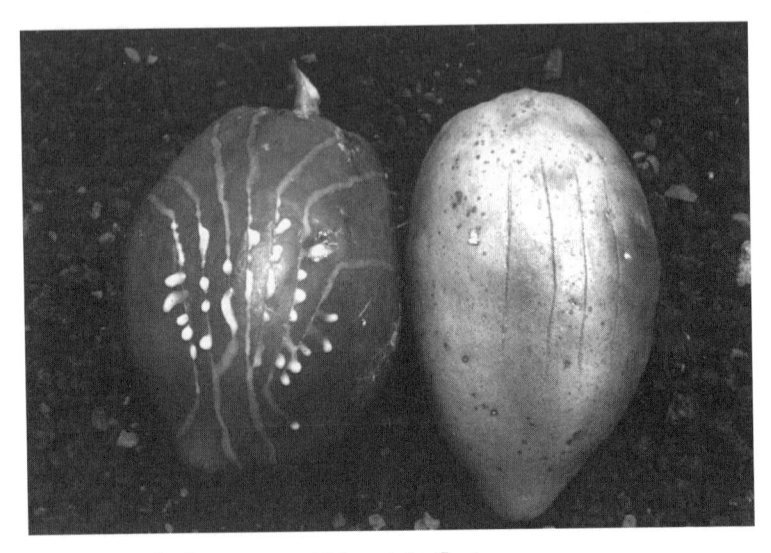

Cut green and yellow papaya with latex juice flowing.

Cancer—Causes and Alternatives

"Cancer is the final stage in years of acting against the laws of nature."

(Helmut Wandmaker)

"Anyone who has an unhealthy lifestyle and eats improperly, spends his whole life preparing for cancer."

(Dr. Kollath, M.D.)

Everyone should know that the battle against cancer is deception for the most part.

(Dr. Linus Pauling, two-time Nobel Prize Laureate)

When patients with cancer ask a doctor what they should eat, they usually get the response: "Eat what you like. There is no diet for cancer." Anyone operated on for cancer usually receives a similar answer: "We have done everything possible for you, keep on living your normal lifestyle, and come back every three to six months for a follow-up examination." As if a check-up could protect someone!

In his very worthwhile book on the revolution in medicine and health, the German Dr. Hans Nieper points out something that I want every cancer patient to take to heart: The human being is affected 24 hours a day by what he or she eats. To claim that diet has no relevance for the control of cancer is absolute nonsense and disqualifies any doctor who says this as an inappropriate partner for the patient who seeks help.[65] Nieper tells of an American doctor who suffered from cancer on the neck and could demonstrate that the tumor grew more quickly after he ate a grilled chicken and drastically decreased in size when he maintained a millet diet.

Can cancer be caused by a faulty diet? According to the German physicians Renner and Canzler: "The initial question as to whether nutrition plays a role in the formation of cancer must be answered with *yes*."[66] Nieper has a similar response: "Diet plays a very significant role in cancer prevention and cancer treatment."[67] In the following I will thoroughly examine this topic and then describe examples of how papaya has been used as a cancer-healing plant for centuries by native peoples, as well as the role it plays in modern medicine.

Toxemia Explained: The True Interpretation of the Cause of Disease is the title of a book by Dr. John H. Tilden, one of the founders of the Natural Hygiene movement in the USA. T. C. Fry's book *Program for Dynamic Health: An Introduction to Natural Hygiene* presents a good introduction to this topic. Toxemia is an overloading of the blood with metabolic poisons. According to John Tilden, illness is a crisis in which these toxins are eliminated. However, in his opinion the actual illness is toxemia.

Tilden and other representatives of Natural Hygiene—including Shelton, Fry, Walker, Marilyn and Harvey Diamond, and Konz and Wandmaker in Germany -believe that we create our own diseases. When we give up our unnatural habits, we can cure any illness as long as our organs have not been irreparably damaged. Accordingly, Tilden interprets illness as the externally recognizable effects of Mother Nature's efforts to free the organism from its rampant toxins.[68] The supporters of Natural Hygiene view illness as the attempt of the ruling life forces to heal.[69] Although disease and death may occur suddenly, they have a long case history. There is only one cause of illness, and there is only one illness that manifests itself in various forms.[70]

According to Tilden, an increasingly intolerable collection of waste matter occurs in the body when stress and exhaustion prevent adequate elimination of harmful substances and toxins from the lungs, intestine, kidneys, and the skin. When the blood and tissue are inundated with damaging substances, he speaks of "toxemia." Disease is always a reaction to an acute crisis or a chronic process. The type and development of the "dis-ease" depends on the individual constitutional tendencies, the personal state of health, and the respective medical treatment. Here is a summary of the stages of an illness:

1. Excessive stimulation (stress)
2. Tension, overexertion
3. Exhaustion

4. Increase of waste matter
5. Toxemia
6. Disease as reaction.

Natural Hygiene sees the cause of all diseases in miserable body chemistry as the result of poor nutrition. The proof of this is the speed with which most health problems disappear when appropriate nutritional changes are made.[71]

The mistakes of our normal modern diet are that it:

- Is too rich in proportion to the amount we eat
- Has too few essential nutrients like vitamins and minerals
- Has too many proteins, fats, starches, and cholesterol
- Has too little natural carbohydrates
- Has too little roughage or fiber
- Has too many refined carbohydrates such as flour, sugar, and alcohol
- Has too many improper spices
- Has too much black tea, coffee, and cola drinks
- Has preservatives that interfere with digestive enzymes
- Destroys the molecular structure of the foods by heating them, and especially by long roasting
- Has additives and other chemicals

Isn't it conspicuous that there are more illnesses in "highly civilized" countries, but these are hardly known to the "primitive" native peoples? Japanese soldiers who survived in the Philippine jungles also escaped from the illnesses of civilization. However, when "primitive natives" eat the "white man's" food, they soon get his diseases as well.

In the summer of 1996, I was in Haiti as a development-aid helper: I was shocked by the health situation of the Haitians—especially those who were doing well economically! In its *World Health Report 1997*, WHO deplored the strong increase in chronic illnesses in underdeveloped countries. This increase can be directly related to adoption of unhealthy Western lifestyles. A lack of physical exercise, the consumption of tobacco and alcohol, and "imbalanced nutrition" in particular are responsible.

According to Natural Hygiene, the entire body's health is dependent upon the quality of the blood and lymph fluid. Because of the toxic substances that get into the blood stream as a result of an unhealthy diet, there is a reduced supply of oxygen to the cells, the normal metabolism is disturbed, and the body's power of resistance toward viral and bacterial attack is reduced. If we restore the correct environment for the cells, the *milieu interieur*, the body can regenerate itself and once again fulfill its normal functions without further help—unless the organs have been destroyed beyond a certain stage. The diseases of modern civilization such as cancer, high blood pressure, migraines, infection of the prostate gland, multiple scleroses (MS), asthma, and many others, disappear and do not return if a healthy lifestyle is assumed.

What is healthy nutrition according to Natural Hygiene? It consists of whole foods from plants: fruit, vegetables, seeds, and sprouts. Even the Bible gives a clear description of the food that is meant for us and is beneficial for us: "And God said, I gave you herbs that bear seeds that grow everywhere on the earth, and every tree whose fruit contains seeds shall serve as food." (Genesis 1.29)

Helmut Wandmaker comments that the cancer problem certainly won't be solved by adding a few minerals like magnesium or selenium to the diet. "When I look at things from the standpoint of natural laws, then we all need minerals and vitamins—the ones that have been discovered and those not yet discovered! And these are adequately present in the correct combination in raw and natural food, which is all that we should be eating. That is, if we weren't constantly destroying our soil ourselves with unbalanced fertilizer, with insecticides and pesticides! First comes a healthy soil, then the healthy plants, and, supported by both, comes the healthy man instead of the civil cripple of today!"[72] Like many others, Wandmaker sees animal protein as one of the reasons for the development of cancer. "Cancerous ulcers have ten times the amount of protein waste than other body tissues, a sign that cancer is substantially related to modern excessive consumption of proteins. Meat has become the most popular 'vegetable'!"[73]

The connection between a high level of meat consumption and intestinal cancer has been established beyond a doubt. In his book

Improving on Pritikin—You Can Do Better!, Ross Horne describes a number of examples of how people with a great diversity of diseases were healed by raw food, sunshine, and rest: among these are AIDS, arthritis, rheumatism, colds, and cancer. Even the great Swedish physician Are Waerland once said that we are not concerned about the illnesses, but with errors; once the errors are corrected, the illnesses will disappear on their own.[74]

Mahatma Gandhi, who suffered from many illnesses as a young man, became interested in naturopathy when he was 32 years old. First he became a vegetarian and then a fruitarian. After six months of eating fruit, he was enthusiastic about the fact that he could work hard for a long time without getting tired. His own experiences and those of the many sick people who ate only fruits according to his instructions convinced him that fruit is the most suitable form of food for human beings.[75]

According to Horne, stress can only cause cancer in a tissue that is already precancerous (one stage before cancer). He believes that a virus—regardless of whether it is a flu or an AIDS virus—is not dangerous for a body that is radiantly healthy. Consequently, a virus cannot be the cause of cancer either. It has been determined that the virus particles found concentrated in blood and tissue of cancer patients, such as herpes, can be found in every individual: they can reproduce themselves now that the immune system is weakened.

There are numerous cancer diets propagating a high proportion of fresh foods and many case examples in which cancer patients were healed through a resolute conversion to raw foods.

Helmut Wandmaker is in extraordinarily good shape, both physically and mentally. At eighty-three years of age, he looks like a sixty-year-old and still has his airplane license, which requires a strict health examination every year. He constantly faxes me thank-you notes from older cancer patients who were healed through raw foods and write that their lives have been saved by Wandmaker's books.

The Persian author A. T. Hovannessian, Wandmaker's great role model, calls cancer the "daughter of the cooking pot" in his book *Raw-Eating*. He recommends more than two pounds of raw fruit every day. "This is enough to maintain a human life, but it is the death sentence for cancer cells."[76] Hovannessian convincingly establishes that cancer cells arise from a deficit of higher nutrients and an excess of these simple substances (formed by denaturization through cooking), which makes the uninhibited growth of cells possible[77].

When we eat fruits, which are rich in highly valuable nutritional components, we can reverse this process and give the cancer cells the valuable abilities that normal cells have and bring them back into balance with the whole. Nutritional pioneers like Kollath, Bircher-Brenner, and Bruker consider fresh food to be a cure for almost all diseases. Wandmaker correctly asks why foods that are recognized as therapy for illnesses are not also resolutely propagated as the ideal standard diet for those who are healthy.

Members of the Seventh Day Adventists in the USA, who almost exclusively eat raw plant foods, are called "the healthiest Americans" because they rarely suffer from diabetes, heart problems, and cancer; they also have a considerably higher life expectancy than the average American. The Mormons also eat many fruits and vegetables with little meat—they have a 30 percent lower occurrence of cancer than people of similar age groups do in the average population.

In addition to slowly digested carbohydrates like millet, rice, and oat flakes, Nieper recommends a cancer diet consisting of many vegetables and fruits. He particularly emphasizes fruits that usually spoil quickly as a result of their wealth of enzymes, including the mango, papaya, pineapple, and banana.[78] On his negative list are meat (maximal 150 g per week!), sugary foods, refined wheat, ready-to-eat-foods, and meals rich in fats. He points out that beta carotene, which occurs abundantly in carrots and papayas, reduces the occurrence of cancer by about 37 percent. Together with other substances, it shows a strong protective effect against the development of cancer. Cancer patients at his hospital—the Paracelsus Klinik Silbersee in Hannover–Langenhagen, Germany—are treated with the corresponding diet, which includes beta carotene, nutritional supplements like magnesium orotat, and bitter-almond extracts (Laetrile or B17). This treatment is apparently very successful: Patients come from all over the world.

In *You CAN Prevent Breast Cancer!*, Harvey Diamond (who wrote the best seller *Fit for Life* with his wife Marilyn) advises patients who have had breast cancer or wish to avoid it to adopt a "mono diet" of raw foods as the most important and strongest instrument in the prevention of cancer. To follow this diet, eat only fresh fruit and/or raw vegetables and their freshly squeezed juices for a day, a week or a month (or a lifetime). In this way, as little energy as possible is used for digestion; instead, it can be used for cleansing and rejuvenating the lymph system[79]. Dr. Renner and Dr. Cantler present a number of cancer diets with a high proportion of raw plant food in their book on nutrition and cancer:

- Max Gerson's cancer therapy of freshly squeezed juices from organically grown fruits, vegetables, leaves (chlorophyll!), and salads.
- The raw vegetable diet according to Bircher-Brenner, in which a high "sunlight value" and maximal effectiveness of raw plant foods play a central role.
- The lacto-vegetable diet according to Werner Kollath in its greatest possible state of biological value: The food should be eaten in its most natural state.
- Karl Windstosser's healing diet with raw fruit or vegetables at every meal.
- Kuhl's lactic-acid diet with a large portion of fruit, salads, raw vegetarian food, and raw vegetable juices.

I particularly want to emphasize the cancer therapy according to Dr. Max Gerson. He was Professor Sauerbruch's assistant and Albert Schweitzer's friend, the latter of which celebrated him as "one of the greatest geniuses in the history of medicine". The Gerson Therapy's intensive nutritional treatment became known through the documentation of how more than 50 cancer patients in an advanced stage were healed. Gerson presented this report to the American Congress. These cases are documented in his book *A Cancer Therapy: Results of 50 Cases and the Cure of Advanced Cancer*. Since his death, Gerson's daughter Charlotte has continued her father's work at Gerson Institute in California.

This therapy fundamentally takes into account the entire organism and forces a total polarity reversal of its dynamics. Gerson not only saw the lack of nutrients as a contributing factor to the development of cancer; he also developed a diet that has an intensive effect on cancerous processes. The basis of the effectiveness and the success of his therapy is the high concentration of pure fresh fruits and vegetables in an easily digestible form as juice (including green leaves), which are taken once an hour. Only organically grown foods are used for this purpose. Gerson denounces how the generally available foods have been negatively effected by fertilizers, pesticides, cesium radiation, preservatives, bleaches and dyes, taste intensifiers, genetic engineering, and much more. He says that if we stay close to nature, its eternal laws will protect us.[80]

The Gerson Therapy is also suitable as a basic therapy for all health disorders, especially chronic illnesses and diseases caused by civilization. The diet essentially consists of much fresh fruits and vegetables. Moreover, it is a low-calorie, salt-free, and low-fat diet.

It takes a great deal of courage to leave the hospital by the back door like Franz Konz—who was scheduled to be operated on for stomach cancer. Instead, he healed himself with raw plant foods, wild herbs, and much exercise. His experiences and therapy instructions are accessible to readers of German in his almost 1600-page book on health, which he wrote primarily for extremely ill people. It will soon be translated into English. The "original medicine" propagated by Konz is not only a remedy for health but also "a world view with possible potential for social change." His book is for all people who are prepared to accept personal responsibility for their bodies, their health, and their future—so that we no longer will have to struggle with cancer in the 21st century.

Gisela Friebel describes in her book about cancer how she won her battle using primarily alkaline raw plant foods. She confirms the old saying: "Only those who heal are right." Since she became afflicted with cancer in 1983, she has held many seminars and lectures, as well as writing ten books, in order to give courage and hope to other cancer patients. I met her personally at one of her talks and she impressed me as having a great deal of vitality.

Another example is Dr. Nolfi, who also cured her own cancer through raw plant foods. From 1945 to 1947, she ran an 80-bed clinic where hundreds of patients were healed of all possible illnesses, including cancer, through a change of diet to fresh fruits and vegetables.

Raw fruits and vegetables are a simple way of allowing the body's own regulatory mechanisms to become effective again. In view of the abundance of health disorders that have been positively influenced through Dr. Kristine Nolfi's fresh-food cures, we can say that it is "malpractice" when nutrition is not used as a basic treatment and preventive. This is especially important after operations to prevent the formation of metastases.

The great American nutrition pioneer Norman Walker, who died of old age at 116, wrote that it is interesting for the layman (but probably not good business for the cancer societies and similar institutes) to learn that people who live exclusively on fresh, raw vegetarian foods complimented with fresh, raw vegetable juices and fruit juices, do not get cancer. He believed that illness is prevented by the cleansing of the body through colon hydrotherapy and enemas, eating an adequate amount of raw plant foods, and drinking a variety of fresh juices.[81]

Papain in Enzyme Therapy against Cancer

Leibold called the South American Indians "the founders of enzyme therapy against cancer" because for centuries they not only have been using the leaves and fruit of the papaya plant for injuries, but also against malignant ulcers. In a similar vein, German author Kurt Allgeier wrote:

"Enzyme treatment of cancer has been used for centuries. The Indians, for example, bound the fruit and leaves of the papaya plant onto severe wounds. They knew that this plant was a great help against burns, infections, and the formation of pus, as well as for malignant tumors. They know from experience that not only did wounds heal and sores disappear, but also the pain diminished as soon as this natural remedy was applied."[82]

The oldest report that I found on the use of papain against cancer was in *The British Medical Journal* of June 16, 1906. W.J. Branch wrote about his success in dissolving tumors by injecting two grams of papain and noted that one of the tumors had to be injected three times with this solution before it dissolved. The author classified papain as a cancer-destroyer and noted that the juice of all parts of the papaw tree appears to have a special "protein-dissolving power." This property is employed in the process of chemical injection (see *Papaya for Backaches—Chemonucleolysis and More* on page 126): The papaya enzyme destroys and dissolves only diseased tissue—healthy tissue is not attacked.

In modern times, cancer therapy with enzymes has only been intensively studied for the past twenty years. It is "on the best road to becoming one of the most important healing processes, without the feared side effects of the customary cancer therapy."[83] Dr. Wolf, the founder of the modern enzyme therapy, discovered that the blood of cancer patients lacks a certain component that prevents the growth of cancer in healthy people. We know that every human being produces between several hundred and 10,000 cancer cells per day; however, they are normally recognized in time and destroyed. Wolf found out that cancer patients lacked a protein-splitting enzyme.

How can a protein-splitting, proteolytic enzyme stop cancer? If the theory that a virus triggers some types of cancer is correct, then the enzyme could take over the important task of being a "virus killer." Living cells can protect themselves against protein-splitting enzymes. But cancer cells can only protect themselves to a certain extent. Their protein materials are different from those of healthy cells, and they only develop enzyme-inhibitory substances after 12 to 48 hours: This is usually enough time for the body's defense system to destroy them.

However, if a cancer cell succeeds in becoming attached to a healthy cell in this race against time, it covers itself with a coat of fibrin. In this way, it disguises itself so that the immune system doesn't recognize it and it begins to grow without inhibition. When too few enzymes are present, they cannot dissolve the sticky fibrin in the blood. The fibrin attaches itself to the white blood cells—which are the defensive cells—and covers them with glue. This prevents them from destroying the cancer cells that have not yet protected themselves with a fibrin network.

Another effect of the protein-splitting enzymes is that they are capable of breaking down the so-called immune complexes that lame the cellular defense. These enzymes then dissolve the immune complexes out of the tissue connection and eliminate them from the organism. In addition, they activate the tumor necrosis factor TNF, a cancer-destroying molecule of the defense system. They also increase the activity of macrophages (large white blood cells) and natural killer cells.

If the body now receives a high-dosage enzyme preparation, it can break down the fibrin on the lymphocytes and the defense system will regain its effectiveness. The coat substance of the tumor cell is removed, and the cell is exposed so that it can be recognized once again as a cancer cell by the body's defense system.

This is particularly important after operations since they increase the body's production of fibrin or when medication or radiation destroys the tumor. In the latter case, the increased fibrin creates favorable conditions for the cancer cells that have been "sown." Although enough practical experience has accumulated by now, clearly emphasizing the necessity of subsequent treatment with enzymes, this approach is seldom incorporated in traditional cancer therapy. It is important to remember that most cancer patients don't die because of the original tumor, but as a result of the tumors formed by metastasis, which could effectively be prevented with enzyme therapy.

Allgeier reports success in local treatment with enzymes such as the "sensational success with pleural carcinoma": instead of a 22 percent chance of recovery, patients with enzyme treatment had a prognosis of 42 percent; for another 42 percent, the tumors reduced to half their size within four months. Similar positive results have been reported for pancreatic cancer, for there has only been a survival rate of one to two percent of the patients for five years. One of the largest cancer clinics in the USA, the Yama Clinic, is conducting a study in which enzymes are placed into solid tumors. "What is impressive about this method is that the destruction and dissolution process carried out by the enzymes stops at the edge of the tumor. No healthy, normal cells are damaged or even destroyed. Enzymes are actually a specific cancer remedy: they destroy the cancer and only the cancer."[84] Leibold therefore sees an important and promising application area for enzyme treatment in preventive and supplementary cancer therapy

Dr. Heinrich Wrba has written a very interesting essay on the topic of enzymes and cancer therapy (in German). Wrba goes so far as to claim: "If we would systematically treat people who have a high risk of getting cancer in a preventive manner—with enzymes, among other things, then we could cut the number of cancer cases in half."[85] To work optimally, enzymes need coenzymes, minerals, trace elements, and vitamins, which we find abundantly in fresh fruits and vegetables.

Carpaine against Cancer?

Professor Chung-Shih Tang, a papaya expert at the University of Honolulu, reports on the effect of carpaine. This is the main alkaloid in the leaves, all the green portions, and the seeds of the papaya. Carpaine not only reduces the blood pressure in a manner similar to digitalis, but is also reported by various authors to have an anti-cancer effect. At a dose of 0.1%, it is said to be effective against cancer of the blood, more commonly referred to as leukemia. However, Professor Tang could not validate these research results in his own experiments with mice.

Dr. McLaughlin of the University of Lafayette (Indiana) also does research on this topic. He has found that papaya leaves dissolve cancer cells.

Case Example: Halima Neumann's Papaya Therapy

German author Halima Neumann reports in both of her books about papaya's therapeutic success against cancer. After several unsuccessful chemotherapy treatments, she was prescribed the freshly squeezed juice of about 2 pounds of green papayas (divided among meals three times a day) by Dr. Kurt Koesel of Maui, Hawaii. The freshly squeezed bitter juice was diluted with half a liter of water and she immediately, but slowly, drank it in sips. In addition to the fruit pulp, the bitter skin and the dark seeds of ripe papaya fruit were also included. For half a year, the weakened cancer patient lived from this liquid. She writes: "The cancer-cell dissolving effect of the white milk under the fruit skin (papain latex) and the enzyme in the seeds initiated the healing of my cancer on the physical level."[86]

After half a year, Halima Neumann began to grate the green papaya fruit and to eat it as raw food—she calls it "papaya herb." In this way, she was able to get her digestive system functioning. She countered the bitter taste of the papaya skin with lemon juice and olive oil. In order to strengthen her weakened body, every day she took 30 grams of spirulina, a protein- and vitamin-rich green algae from chemical-free soda water. After one year of "papaya therapy," no more cancer cells could be found in her bladder and uterus.

In addition to the effect of the green papaya and the seeds of the ripe fruit, Halima Neumann also learned how important a new emotional orientation is for a cancer illness: "After many healing crises during the first six months, I finally began to discover my true self with a clear consciousness. In the beginning, I placed my entire hopes for recovery in natural healing substances and help from the outside. After the repeated crises had passed, there was an enormous improvement. However, complete healing was delayed until I realized that it was also necessary to change something in my consciousness. In this way, I discovered how divine love works with the inner healer and the long-desired recovery took place. I finally felt centered—healthy, whole, and secure!"[87]

Today, after more than seventeen years, Halima Neumann is considered to be fully healed and shares her knowledge through books and seminars. Enthusiastic about the beneficial, healthy properties of the green papaya as a preventive and universal healing remedy for chronic health disorders and immune weakness, the health consultant began searching for a suitable site on the Canary Islands. She now has found an appropriate piece of property on the Island of La Palma, where a self-help center is planned. People with poor health can regenerate using the papaya therapy and also learn a new, healthier lifestyle and diet at the seminars (also in English, on request.)

The deacidification, anti-cancer, and anti-fungal treatments at the planned center will also be open to anyone who wants to contribute work to the project instead of paying money. The land is about 830 feet above the sea with a fantastic panoramic view, only twelve minutes by car from the black lava beach "Charco Verde." Financial backers are still being sought for the building plans and urbanization for cultivating papaya and aloe vera in a mixed culture. If they wish, they can also apply their loan toward free seminar visits or living in the green garden of recuperation.

Halima Neumann reports in her cancer book about the papaya therapy that was first successfully used in the USA and now in Mexico near the American border. The successor of Harold Manner, who wrote a number of books on the topic, treats cancer patients with Laetrile from the apricot pit and papaya latex at the "Manner Clinic" in Tijuana, Mexico. Laetrile, also called vitamin B17 or amygdalin, can be obtained from apricot pits, almond nuts, papaya, and many other plants. When these bitter almond substances release cyanide and benzaldehyde because of an enzyme reaction, the cancer cells supposedly die while the healthy cells are not influenced.

(Translator's note: The American Cancer Society has found no evidence that Laetrile alone has a significant effect on cancer. Although 75,000 Americans are believed to have used it, only two cases were judged to have experienced complete recovery and four a partial recovery from a total of 62 reported cases. An excessive dosage can result in neuromuscular weakness, respiratory distress, nerve degeneration, and death.)

Harold Manner, who worked at the Loyola University in Chicago, reportedly attained a success rate of 68 percent in the shrinking of tumors with a special anti-cancer diet and therapy. According to Halima Neumann, his success with the colon hydrotherapy (intestinal cleansing, for explanation see *Intestinal Health* on page 87), large vitamin doses (especially a precursor of vitamin A, vitamin B complex, vitamin C, and vitamin B17), the thymus extract levamisol, and interferon.

Information about further clinics that work with Laetrile are available from the Cancer Control Society (213/663-7801). Manuel Gomez de la Maza, professor at the University of Havana, also claimed success in healing cancer patients with Laetrile and papaya latex, the white milk that seeps out from beneath the skin of the green fruit.

During her period of healing on Hawaii, Halima Neumann met with Dr. Koesel and Dr. Ray, as well as countless patients who were healed through their papaya therapy.

The Papaya as Australia's Cancer-Healing "Remedy"

Harald Tietze's small book *Kombucha: The Miracle Fungus*, which suggests the papaya as a way of healing cancer, had previously received relatively little attention. However, when Ruediger Schlegel wrote an article about the "thousand-year-old cancer-healing plant of the Aborigines" in the German magazine *Bio* at the beginning of 1997, based on scientific proof by Dr. McLaughlin of Purdue University (West Lafayette, Indiana), an avalanche of questions was sent to the publisher. The "Papaya Super Concentrate" that he distributes has apparently developed into a best seller for healing practitioners, naturopathic doctors, and their patients.

However, since it has been proved that papayas have only been known to Australia for the past 200 years, we are not dealing with a "thousand-year-old Aboriginal recipe" (Schlegel's words). Secondly, the study by Dr. McLaughlin, whom I questioned in this regard, refers to the "long leaf papaw" and not the "Carica papaya," which is known in Australia as "papaw." The Latin name for the "long leaf papaw" is Asimina longifolia, and it is not even distantly related to the "Carica papaya." The "long leaf papaw" is a bush from the Mississippi Delta. Any "scientific proof" fades away in the light of this fact. However, Dr. McLaughlin told me that he had received a few papaya leaves from Harald Tietze and had the first indications of a possible related cancer-inhibiting effect. A short time ago, he assigned his students to this project, but final results are not yet available.

Perhaps the "Papaya Super Concentrate" does have an effect on cancer; however, there is no proof of this as of yet. I will remain in contact with Dr. McLaughlin and perhaps report on his experience in a future book. In Australia, the "Papaya Super Concentrate" has been available for about three years in natural food stores. Harald Tietze sent me a positive patient report. But the man was also given radiation therapy for one month. He no longer has lung cancer and has been relatively free of complaints for the past three years.

"Papaya 7 Super Concentrate," which contains more papaya leaves, is a new development from Kombucha House, makers of the "Papaya Super Concentrate." The original Aborigine recipe was rediscovered by

Frank Sheldon of eastern Australia and optimized by José Perko, an Australian skilled in naturopathy. Then it was developed into this product. Cancer patients have also had good experiences with the "Papaya & Guava" concentrate. Sea minerals with papaya, a remedy that has a similar effect, are also available as a preventative nutritional supplement. For more information see *Resources* on page 207. Organically grown dried and fermented papaya leaves, with which the original Aborigine recipe can be prepared, are also available. I have included the Aborigine recipe in *The Papaya as a Healing Plant of the Aborigines* on page 146.

Harald Tietze replied to questioning, that one could also eat unripe papaya with core instead of taking leaves or simply eat the fruit raw. He mentions something similar in his kombucha book "In areas, where no papaw-trees grow, half-ripe papaw fruit is also used. The fruit is eaten together with the skin and seeds." It is recommended that they be prepared as "papaya herb" (see *Recipes for the Kitchen* on page 160) because of the bitter taste. I can recommend Harald Tietze's book on papaya "Papaya (Pawpaw), the Medicine Tree", see *Bibliography*.

The Australian doctor John Wittman Ray has made a video on "Body Electronics" in which he speaks about the papaya's healing power in cases of cancer (see *Resources* on page 207).

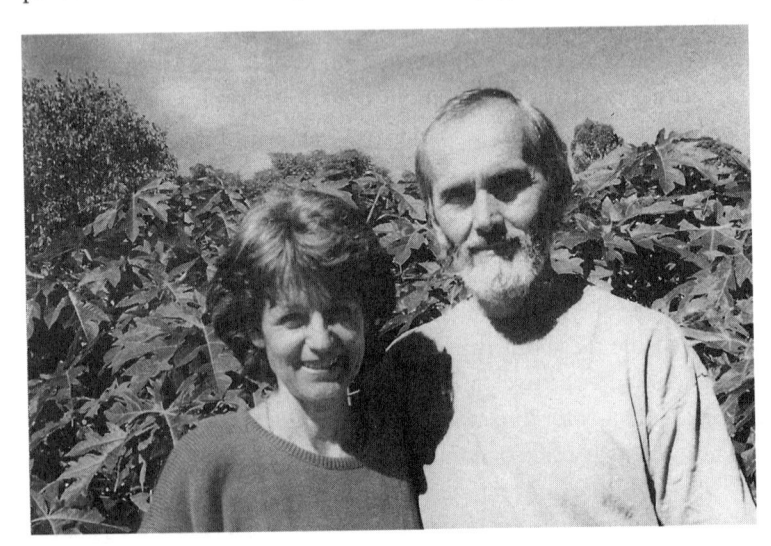

Veronika and José Perko—founders of "Kombucha House"

Allergies—
When the "Barrel" is Full!

The German society of neurodermatitis sufferers speaks of two million afflicted in that country and estimates the number of unknown cases to be equally high. There are a total of 25 million people suffering from allergies in Germany (total population: 78 million) with a rising tendency. The rate of increase for neurodermatitis alone is seven percent or 140,000 new occurrences per year. If the development continues at this same rate, every German citizen will have an allergy within ten years!

The subject of "allergies" is complex, and the problem is attaining explosive dimensions. Already one-fifth of the US-children suffer from nutritional allergies and other allergies. Many physicians and healing practitioners recommend that everything white be eliminated from the diet. This includes all white flour products and possibly even wheat itself, sugar, and animal proteins such as milk products. Flour and milk are the foods that most often trigger allergies. Wheat is an overbred grain: Many people who are allergic to wheat (even from organic cultivation) use spelt, the original form. Even synthetic additives that start with the letter "E" should be avoided. The dangerous thing about allergies is that they may develop into asthma after a few years.

Babies should be breastfed as long as possible—a period of one year is good. After this, they shouldn't eat any milk products and other "foreign" animal proteins. There are enough high-quality proteins in vegetables, nuts, seeds, and fruits! Many ethnic groups on this planet eat no milk products and enjoy the best of health.

It's no wonder that we react to a few of these unnatural foods with allergies. Our organism already is busy enough with environmental toxins and synthetic materials. We never know when "the barrel is full" and begins to run over in the form of an allergy! Consequently, we should attempt to obtain the most natural form of food that has been grown organically without pesticides, insecticides, fungicides, and fertilizer and processed as little as possible. It is also advisable to live and work in natural surroundings.

Wandmaker and other supporters of Natural Hygiene make toxemia, the poisoning of the body and waste accumulation within it, responsible for the increasing allergy and asthma problems. "When the inner organs—especially the large purification factory of the liver and the last filtering organ, the kidney—can no longer manage to eliminate the constantly accumulating waste substances normally through bowel movements, urine, and lungs, the largest excretory organ, our skin, is used to maintain the life of the organism."[88] Wandmaker recommends that we revert to a 100-percent raw plant diet: "then allergies, acne and neurodermatitis disappear within a few weeks."

Natural Hygiene maintains that those suffering from allergies are not ill but so healthy that they are still in possession of vital defensive powers against the substances that make us sick. I would like to share my own experience in this regard: Since I eliminated animal proteins from my diet years ago, I have become so sensitive to them that I can't eat them. My (identical) twin sister is able to eat milk products and still has no problems with them. But in contrast to her, I am never sick: I have no colds and no arthritis in the shoulders. Perhaps those who suffer from allergies are not the sick people but the "healthy" ones who apparently seem to tolerate everything? In this respect, it is interesting to note that those with allergies have a much lower rate of cancer than the average population.

One of the main causes of increasing allergies is certainly the "protein garbage" that most people have in their intestines. "Particularly those who suffer from allergies such as neurodermatitis are affected by a protein metabolic disturbance. This is combined with hyperacidic tendencies in the small intestine and the passing of large-molecule proteins into the blood."[89]

A papaya treatment can help in this case: Eat a papaya every day if possible, preferably together with its papain-containing seeds, or take an enzyme preparation containing papain! The papaya enzymes break down the "protein garbage" in the intestine, heal perforated intestinal walls, normalize the imbalanced intestinal flora, and degrade the immune complexes. Undigested food molecules are treated as foreign bodies in the blood. The lymphocytes of the immune system produce antibodies that attach themselves to these molecules in order to identify them. The white immune cells then consume these immune complexes. However, if there are too many, they form deposits in the muscles, skin, brain, lungs, arteries, and other body areas. This leads to inflammations, pain, and signs of degeneration in the afflicted area.

By fighting these "nutritional poisons," the body often loses its capacity to defend itself successfully against viruses and bacteria. The nutritional allergy can lead to complex problems: asthma, diarrhea, colitis, rashes, rheumatism, and multiple sclerosis. Papaya enzymes free our stomach and intestine walls from parasites, bacteria, and fungi (compare with *Intestinal Health* on page 87, *Papaya Gets Rid of Worms* on page 122, and *Papaya Combats Fungal Disease* on page 116).

Moreover, the vitamins in the papaya strengthen our weakened immune system. In any case —at least for a while—we should eliminate those foods from our diet that cause an allergic reaction. To support our immune system, we should eat as many fresh fruits and vegetables as possible, get much exercise in clean air, reduce stress, and build up our resistance by taking cold showers (or alternating hot and cold showers).

After three months of this program, we can reintroduce a food that previously caused immunoglobulin reactions since the memory of lymphocytes only lasts from two to three months. To activate self-healing powers, cleanse the body, and conquer stress, I also recommend that you learn Authentic Reiki. This is a method that even children can learn. People suffering from the worst asthma attacks every night have eliminated their symptoms within six weeks by using it.

Papaya—
Help for Colds and Flu

Viruses cause colds and flu. An influenza infection or a cold is an acute illness of the respiratory system, which is often accompanied by fever. The influenza virus types A, B, and C cause a genuine flu.

People in India traditionally use an extract from the mashed seeds of the papaya and vinegar, which increases perspiration, for colds and flu. Cooking the young leaves like vegetables is reported to fight against fever in the early stage of the flu. Papayas prevent colds by abundantly supplying us with vitamin C and fill up the body's enzyme supply so that we are well protected against the attack of viruses. A person who eats many fresh fruits and vegetables, or even primarily raw plant foods, won't catch colds very often, if at all.

Professor Max Wolf, the founder of modern enzyme therapy, carried out a long-term study with Canadian soldiers. They received a suitable enzyme mixture as a preventive measure. "Afterwards, two-thirds of those who were usually sick with the flu or colds several times a year remained healthy. The remaining participants became only slightly ill. Not a single serious case of the flu occurred."[90] No other preventive treatment (which is without any side effects) has demonstrated such good results.

When an organism has enough enzymes, it cannot become infected because every virus entering the organism is immediately attacked and killed. Those who have already caught the flu or a cold can also profit from taking the enzymes, which destroy the "descendants" of the virus formed within infected cells. If an infection already exists, its duration is shortened: The cell debris is broken down more quickly, viscid mucus in the respiratory system is dissolved, and the symptoms are relieved.

Papaya—Help for the Heart!

Cardiovascular diseases are the primary cause of death in America. Every year more than 500,000 people die of them in the USA. Vasoconstriction leads to high blood pressure and, above all, damages the heart and kidneys. Researchers assume that an enzyme shortage exists at the beginning of arteriosclerosis. This is because the fat-splitting biocatalyst is involved in preventing the formation of deposits in the arteries or the breakdown of existing deposits.

Wandmaker recommends a heart-protection diet: "Eat the ideal food—raw plant foods, preferably fruit. Even if a compromise is necessary, don't give up eating two meals of uncooked fruits and vegetables every day."[91] The constriction of the capillaries because of calcium deposits is primarily due to a lack of vitamin C. Consequently, the best capillary protection is raw, whole food with its high contents of enzymes and coenzymes. Enzyme preparations are recommended for all stages of arteriosclerosis, for the follow-up treatment of heart attacks and strokes, and for less critical circulatory problems. "Enzymes can be taken as a preventive treatment, preferably for several weeks at a time and a number of times a year, in order to "clean out" the arteries. Continuous intake isn't a problem either. This preventive health treatment should be started, at the latest, when you turn 40!"[92]

Ross Horne says that arteriosclerosis can even be reversed at an advanced stage if the diet is changed! The same goes for diseases that are related to it. The great enzyme researcher Max Wolf discovered that enzyme mixtures combat artery deposits. After taking enzymes himself and giving them to patients, he established that the blood lipid concentration sank conspicuously three to five hours afterwards.

More recent research has shown that eating both unripe and ripe papayas reduces the risk of arteriosclerosis, strokes, and heart attacks. The alkaloid carpaine found in the papaya lowers the blood lipid concentration and cholesterol levels. It can also regenerate a hardened fatty liver. With the appropriate diet, it is possible to break down the cholesterol that has accumulated in the arteries.

Papaya against Inflammation

An inflammatory process accompanies many illnesses. The papaya enzyme papain supports the body in healing inflammations and prevents them from getting out of control. Papain thins the blood, breaks down poisonous substances in the focus of the inflammation, and prevents the formation of pathological immune complexes that lead to new inflammations and interfere with the body's own defense system. Accompanying pains are reduced at their source when the enzymes dissolve the harmful substances irritating the sensitive nerve endings.

The South American Indians supported the healing process by placing slices of papaya and mashed seeds on infected and inflamed skin. Today, we can use ointments containing papain, as well as taking enzyme tablets internally, to support healing processes. Sometimes after treating wounds or sores with enzyme ointments, a small amount of bleeding occurs. "This can be explained by the liquefaction of dead tissue and is advantageous for healing."[93]

Dr. Kunze in Berlin has been studying the effect of papain on the dissolution of immune-complexes, which are networks of several antigens. In the process, he has proved that papain helps the body to repel invading germs by catching them with specific antibodies. The formation of too many antibody aggregates (immune complexes) in an excessive immune reaction can be dangerous for the body because they can develop into new infection centers themselves and slow down the body's defenses. Immune illnesses such as rheumatism, multiple sclerosis, or even chronic infections may develop. Too many immune complexes have also been found in the case of cancer.

Dr. Kunze discovered that even very low concentrations of papain could prevent the formation of too many immune complexes. Papain is present in many enzyme medications and can help to dissolve mucous masses resulting from bronchitis and sinusitis. When antibiotics are administered, the mucous membrane often reacts too strongly; this doesn't occur with enzyme preparations.

All types of inflammations—including bladder infections, chronic ovarian inflammations, and pneumonia—have been effectively treated with combination enzyme preparations. "Enzymes do not function like antiphlogistic agents, which inhibit inflammation, but support everything that helps limit the damage and stimulate the formation of new and healthy tissue."[94] In the medicine of India, the papaya is eaten for stomach and intestinal infections and the South American Indians also use the curative power of the papaya in this manner for the quick healing of inflammations (see *The Ethno-Medicine of Native Peoples* on page 134).

Papaya Combats Fungal Disease (Mycosis)

Wolfgang Spiller writes: "A new era has dawned in medicine—the age of mycosis."[95] He blames this on the use of antibiotics, contraception with the pill, and chemical therapy, as well as "the miserable education of doctors and healing practitioners." Apparently, the weakening of the immune system (for example, through environmental poisons) has lead to an epidemic spread of fungi or mycosis. Certain fungi, such as *Candida albicans,* cause mycosis. Infection can occur through laundry, towels, or dishes, among other things.

Not all people are equally "receptive" to fungi. Like plants, they grow best where they find optimal conditions. Lymphatic people who eat a poor diet are particularly endangered. Those with enough vitamins, enzymes, trace elements, and an overall diet of alkali-forming food are better protected (see *Help against Acidosis* on page 77). Every disturbance of the immune system lowers the threshold for unwanted fungus growth. Concentrated carbohydrates such as sweets, soft drinks, and cake are ideal "food" for fungi. A deadly process can develop on the basis of a harmless virus or fungal infection.

Christine Heideklang points out the increased number of fungal infections in newborns and relates them to the mother's lack of selenium. It's also apparent that newborns can already become infected with *Candida* fungus in the birth canal. People who suffered as children from cradle cap and later from psoriasis are particularly receptive to fungal infections. Ulla Kinon asks in her German-language book on mycosis why we have such an extreme increase in such an illness at this time. She also gives the answer: "Mycosis is always a sure indication of an energy deficiency or orthomolecular (nutritional) deficit, of an acid-alkali shift, allergies, and chronic poisoning..." In her opinion, mycosis always results from a disturbed pH value, whether of the skin or the inner organs (also see *Help against Acidosis* on page 77).

When there is a fungus infection, the fungi eventually choke out the healthy intestinal bacteria. This means that food can no longer be utilized completely. A general state of immune weakness arises, which causes an even more extensive fungal attack. External mycosis of the skin and mucous membranes thrives in a moist environment with pH values that are too acidic. All fungi prefer an organism with unnatural lifestyles, which has unfortunately become the normal state today. Many experts estimate the presence of fungi in 70 to 90 percent of the overall population.

Food definitely has a large influence on our "receptivity to fungi." The German healing practitioner Ulla Kinon has found that a person whose life force is weakened by environmental influences, stress, and false nutrition is afflicted significantly more frequently and intensely by mycosis: "Just as we absorb positive life force with natural, sun-warmed foods, we reduce our vital energy—unnoticed and unconsciously—to the limits of viability with radiated and denatured products."[96]

It is interesting to know that pathogenic fungi prefer sick and dead tissue in human and animal bodies as a host organ and source of food. The fungi that infest the inner organs and mucous membrane are often identical with those of the skin. They change their habits when they wander from external points to the interior because an afflicted person has a weak defensive system. For this reason, we not only find mycosis on the visible skin, but far too often in the inner organs as well. All of a sudden we discover that an atypical bronchitis is mycosis, and the painful flatulence of an infant disappears quickly after effective mycotic therapy.

For chronic digestive problems, skin problems, allergies, and complaints that are therapy resistant, a pathological *Candida* colonization should be taken into consideration. The metabolic poisons that the fungus pours into the blood stream can result in numerous symptoms including migraines, depressions, loss of libido, neurodermatitis, flatulence, heartburn, and colic.

In the magazine *Gesundes Leben* (Healthy Life), February 1993, it is reported that in studies of schools, *Candida* has been found in 80 percent of all German children examined. It is possible that lack of concentration and insufficient interest in learning, as well as susceptibility to infection, are a direct result. The American physicist Steven Rochiltz (author of *Allergies and Candida with the Physicist's Rapid Solution*) discovered that the *Candida* fungus develops the poisonous gas acetaldehyde, which destroys the messenger materials in the corpus callosum, the nerve bundle fibers that connect the two brain halves with each other.

Here are further symptoms that are associated with a *Candida* attack:
- Aggressive moods
- Asthma
- Bronchitis

- Diarrhea or constipation
- Fatigue
- Gingivitis
- Headaches
- Hormonal imbalances
- Infections
- Low blood sugar
- Neurodermatitis
- Sleep disturbances
- Sugar addiction
- Thyroid gland disturbances
- Vaginal excretions
- Weight gain

Ulla Kinon describes the typical course of the disease: "The symptoms of flatulence and pain are intensified because the fungi ferment carbohydrates and form alcohol, gases, and an infection of the intestinal membrane. The gases swell the stomach. The intestine presses against the nearby nerves and impedes the heart and respiration. Alcohol strains the liver, which must degrade and excrete it together with the putrefying toxins that have formed. The fungus slowly crowds out the healthy intestinal flora. The nutrients are not utilized by the body, resulting in a general weakening of the defenses. This in turn is cause for a new fungi attack."[97]

The *Candida* fungus spreads primarily on the intestinal membrane; for example, this occurs when useful intestinal bacteria are killed by antibiotics. Not only medications such as contraceptive pills and cortisone, but also meat and eggs as well as milk products from fattened animals with high concentrations of antibiotics, have a destructive effect on the intestinal flora. Today, even babies are born with *Candida;* their mothers were usually infected with *Candida* without knowing it.

Halima Neumann writes that treating the symptoms with antimycotic agents does not attack the problem at its roots. "By 98 percent of 2,500 cases in Dr. Felix Perger's practice in Austria, there was a relapse after a few months when only an antimycotic medication was used without rebuilding the intestinal flora and changing the diet."

She recommends colon hydrotherapy or intestinal cleansing and reestablishing the intestinal flora with foods that have a low percentage of carbohydrates and sugars.

If you decide on a thorough intestinal cleaning by colon hydrotherapy, you can cut the relatively expensive costs in half by eating 30 to 40 gray to black papaya seeds in the morning on an empty stomach with a cup of water for 6 to 8 weeks before the treatment. If the fruit is not too sweet, it can also be eaten. Eating grated, unripe papaya together with a quarter teaspoon of pulverized seeds intensifies the effect. In this manner, the crust of the intestinal walls can be removed step by step and the hardened deposits can be softened. After successful intestinal cleaning and a fungus-free diet, no special steps are necessary to reestablish the symbiosis.

Halima Neumann recommends the natural fungal killers pau d'arco tea, garlic, and horseradish for light fungal attacks and as a preventive remedy; for intensive fungal attack, use grapefruit seed extract, myrrh, or Dr. Clark's treatment (see her new cancer book).

Mycosis indicates a deep disturbance of the entire person. If you disregard the emotional level, you will not attain a lasting cure because we are a unity of body mind, and soul. Mycosis attacks of a specific organ indicate something that has not been accepted or mastered. Fungal invasion forces the unsolved problem into our consciousness.

Moreover, fungal invasion always has something to do with defective self-confidence and occurs when the soul's demands for growth and change remain unheard. We can either see crises and difficult situations as a challenge or escape into illness because of a negative, pessimistic attitude toward life—the glass is half empty instead of half full.

Here are a few tips:
- Eating papayas helps reestablish the acid-alkali equilibrium and remove the (acidic) environment supporting fungal growth in the intestine. Dr. Renate Collier writes in her book on intestinal cleansing that even feeding cows' milk to babies and small children disturbs the intestinal flora and makes it easy for fungi and other health disturbances to occur.

- Fasting to clean away the waste deposits can be dangerous in cases of *Candida* because the fungus wanders through the intestinal wall in the absence of food and can release its poisonous metabolites into the blood steam. Other organs may be damaged in this way.
- In order to "starve" a *Candida* fungus, a diet with a low percentage of carbohydrates and adequate proteins—on a plant basis—is recommended. In order to remove the dead fungus and metabolic deposits, use a papaya granulate (can be ordered from Papaya John) or grated, fresh green papaya. Psyllium seed husks can also be taken to remove intestinal poisons. The taste of these remedies can be improved with lemon juice, applesauce, and/or olive oil. In a letter to me, Halima Neumann wrote that: "Fresh, green papaya juice from green, unripe fruits is the best cleansing agent for cells and arteries. It helps to break down all inflammation processes, tumors, ulcers, etc."
- Natural roughage and fiber materials are very important for the removal of fungal metabolic deposits. For this purpose, the green papaya can be used as a vegetable like carrots (raw or cooked) and can be included with every food combination. For lunch as an anti-*Candida* diet, Halima Neumann recommends "papaya herbs" from a granulate or freshly grated green papayas with a sour-tasting apple. When there is a *Candida* attack, the pituitary gland and enzyme activity are usually weakened. It may be that the raw vegetables and fruits are not tolerated well, leading to flatulence. An applesauce made from grated raw apples without the skin and papaya herbs is an easy-to-digest alternative.
- Drinking a ten-percent solution of a hot-water papaya extract has also proved beneficial.
- A good opportunity for improving self-esteem and problem-solving abilities is to talk with an experienced therapist or learn a technique for personal growth and transformation (such as Authentic Reiki).

Papaya Gets Rid of Worms

Even Aristotle was interested in parasites. Since he didn't have a microscope, he believed that intestinal parasites were the result of spontaneous generation. He considered the small life forms to be the result of special circumstances. Hippocrates thought that worms and other parasites could be passed from one human generation to the next.

Papaya, especially the green fruit and the seeds of the ripe fruit, as well as the leaves, have been used as a preventive and therapeutic remedy against worms in man and animals for centuries in the nations of the South Sea.

Especially in the tropics and sub-tropics, there are many dangerous amebas, hook worms, pinworms, ascarids, trypanosomes, and other pests, which reproduce themselves through millions of eggs. A few of these parasites suck blood from the mucous membrane of the intestine; others cause infections, abscesses, and sores, venturing as far as the liver. Sometimes the afflicted person or animal dies of the direct or indirect consequences.

Infestation with worms is not considered harmless. Small pinworms can cause an unpleasant itching in the anus, and thousands of them may be found in the large intestinal loops. Ascarids (roundworms) live in the small intestine. In addition, there are *Trichurida* (whipworms) and many other intestinal parasites. They frequently lead to severe health problems. In many types of worm infestation, the afflicted person's blood composition may show typical changes – "eosinophilic". Blood deficiencies, liver damage, and other problems may be the consequences.

The Swiss naturopathic physician and author Bogel assumes that at least 20 to 30 percent of all people in Western Europe are infected with intestinal parasites. He estimates the percentage in hot climates to be 50 to 80 percent. According to the publications of the World Health Organization, WHO, every fourth person has ascarids. Every fifth person is probably infested with one of the two types of hookworms. If the trypanosomes and other intestinal parasites are included, Vogel reaches the assumption that possibly every third person is infected with intestinal parasites. That means about two billion people worldwide!

All small organisms "eat along with" their host, weakening him or her in the process. Moreover, there is the additional strain of more or less toxic metabolic products. These poisons burden the entire organism and damage the liver in particular. There are other very small parasites that can be dangerous to us. For example: flagellates, lamblia, salmonella, and amebas. Lamblia, or small ciliate, which used to be native to warmer countries, often take up residence in our intestines. In some parts of Europe, about 10 to 20 percent of the population is afflicted by them. The number is about twice as high in the USA, with an increasing tendency as a result of increased travel. Children are more strongly affected than adults are.

The effects of parasite attack on children are often dramatic. Vogel: "Children who are infested by ascarids or pinworms usually suffer from typical symptoms such as chlorosis, anemia, loss of appetite, an addiction to sweets, a reduction in learning abilities and receptivity, distraction, lack of energy, and often a strong disturbance of the emotional equilibrium."[98] Accordingly, it's possible that pale children who are always tired and in a bad mood have worms. They should be examined for this possibility. Other signs are nervousness, a lack of patience, constant brooding, shadows under the eyes, and tossing and turning in bed.

In the tropics, one can catch bilharziasis, a very dangerous tropical disease, by swimming in fresh water. Parasites transmit it by boring through healthy skin; subsequently, white worms develop in the inner organs such as the kidneys, liver, lungs, and heart. Even a single footbath in fresh water can lead to this disease. Tourists to Egypt, East Africa, and South Africa are at particular risk. The milky juice of an unripe papaya should immediately be applied to areas that itch.

Another source of danger in the countries of Southeast Asia is raw fish. By eating it, people can contract the fish tapeworm *Diphylobothrium latum* and other dangerous parasites. Because they eat water nuts, which are fertilized with human excrement, forty percent of the population of south China and Hong Kong are thought to have giant intestinal leeches. These parasites can grow to be two centimeters thick and five centimeters long. A further leech living in the small intestine (like "*Echinostoma ilocanum*") is found in dogs and rats on Java and the Philippines.

In his health books, Dr. A. Vogel recommends eating one papaya leaf the size of a half dollar, chewing a teaspoon of the black seeds, or taking two tablets of "Papayasan" after every meal in southern countries, and especially in the tropics and subtropics, as a preventive remedy. The papain contained therein digests all the parasites that infest the large and small intestine. An additional benefit of these precautions is protection against infections.

Another possibility is eating a small amount of seeds together with the ripe fruit, so that they don't taste so bitter. This outstanding remedy against worms also breaks down amebas as long as they are in the intestine.

Dr. Sepp Hannak calls the whipworm *(Trichurida)* the "apparently most common parasite of human beings" in his German-language article on trichuriasis. According to his information, infestation is very widespread in central and southern Italy and has reached up to 100 percent of the population in some areas. In Germany, the occurrence of whipworms is often more common than that of human roundworm: Studies in the town of Baden indicate that 25 percent of the school children are infected; in Kiel, 11 percent are infected with whipworm and 8.2 percent with human roundworm. The mature members of the species bore into the intestinal mucous membrane and suck the blood of their host organism. The symptoms can appear similar to those of tuberculosis: Navel colics, personality changes, headaches, lack of appetite, pains similar to rheumatism in the joints, tiredness, and pain caused by pressure in the lower abdomen can occur.

Bodo J. Baginski and Shalila Sharamon (authors of *The Healing Power of Grapefruit Seed)* warn that 25 percent of the state of New York's population is infested with intestinal parasites and that about half of all Americans are infected at some point in their lives. (Similar large-scale studies have not yet been done in Europe.) Dr. Hulda Clark has found that intestinal and liver leeches can cause a countless number of types of cancer, and Dr. Steven Rochlitz writes in his book *Allergies and Candida* that more than 50 percent of the water supply in the USA is infested with *Giardia lamblia*, a type of parasite.

The natives of South and Central America have used the juice containing enzymes of various fig tree types—*Ficus carica*—and the melon tree *(Carica papaya)* against worms. American literature emphasizes the almost specific effect of these enzyme-containing juices.

In conclusion, I would like to mention another basic perspective. In his book on raw foods, Helmut Wandmaker writes that anthropoid apes normally remain free of parasites as long as they are given their natural food. Only after they are fed with cooked food, do they get parasites, for example, on the skin and in the bowels. He sees "degenerate," denatured food as responsible for the change. A few tips: Vogel recommends that intestinal parasites be fought with the papaya seeds: chew about 10 papaya seeds (or eat one tablespoon of the seeds) every day for three weeks; after a pause for three week, repeat the treatment since natural remedies like papaya kill the worms but not the eggs. Repeat this process until no more worms can be seen. The method can also be applied to animals. Vogel recommends using this treatment once a year as a preventive cure.

- The best part of the treatment is that the papaya has no side effects. Many other medications involve large health risks. An example of a medication containing papain is "Papayasan". It can be used without risk on adults who are frail, children, and pregnant women.
- Glaesel recommends as an alternative that one eat a few raw carrots on an empty stomach mornings and evenings to get rid of pinworms *(Enterobius vermicularis)*. Carrots contain an ethereal oil that has antibacterial and vermifugal (Latin *vermis* = worm and *fugare* = drive away) effects. To eliminate ascarids, it is necessary to only eat about two pounds of raw carrots during the course of 24 hours. It's best to eat this amount grated.
- You can also use grapefruit seed extract to get rid of certain parasites.

Papaya for Backaches—Chemonucleolysis and More

> *"Never forget, gentlemen, that even a successful operation only proves you didn't know how to heal a disease."*
>
> (Professor Hyrtl, Vienna)

Since the 1960s, there has been an alternative to operations for slipped disks and pain in the vicinity of the lumbar vertebra: chemonucleolysis, in which chymopain obtained from the papaya is injected into the nucleus pulposus between the intervertebral disks. The possible side effects of this method usually occur less frequently and are less serious than those of a disk operation, in which deformity or even paraplegia can occur. Spinal column operations produce major complications about ten times more frequently than the injection technique does.

Since ancient times, humans have been plagued by degenerative maladies of the spinal column resulting from erect posture. Even running birds, such as the ostrich, suffer from such problems. The book of Genesis describes the illness of Jacob, a nephew of Abraham: Jacob apparently suffered from sciatica complaints. Examination of bones from the late Neolithic has revealed that almost half of them show deteriorative disorders of the spinal column. However, there are also doctors who do not view back problems as an unavoidable disease of wear, but explain them as resulting from our acid-forming diets (see *Help against Acidosis* on page 77) and widespread lack of sufficient physical exercise.

In his book on rheumatism, Dr. Klaus Hoffmann writes: "Immobilization, inactivity, and lack of exercise are the greatest factors leading to joint and bone damages." Hoffmann has found that even a narrowed joint cavity documented by X-rays can be broadened with good nutrition and physical exercise.

Degenerative phenomena can even be observed in four-year-old children, and after the 30th year of life almost everyone has back problems. "The number of disk operations for patients in the group from 20 to 30 years of age has increased enormously during the past decade."[99] The youngest patients operated on for a slipped disk were between 9 and 13 years of age. When we sit, 980 to 1,800 newton exert pressure on the disk, and when we carry heavy objects this may reach up to 2,200 newton. Physical exercise is important to improve the nutrition of the intervertebral tissue since fluid flows in and out when we move. Many people have too little exercise. Excess weight and poor posture intensify these problems.

Especially between the ages of 30 and 50, the fiber structure of the disk tissue is increasingly worn down. As a result, the disk is less able to act as a shock absorber and the vertebral column is excessively stressed. Tears occur in the cartilage plate and spinal column begins to stiffen. Excessive strain and irritation of the spinal column ("lumbar syndrome") result in arthritis and additional back problems. Changes due to aging primarily effect the lower lumbar disks. The lumbar sacrum disks are the first to show intensive wear. Two-thirds of all back problems involve the lumbar vertebrae region, almost one-third affect the neck, and only one percent is located in the thoracic spine. The clinical symptoms of the lumbar disk syndrome extend from slight backaches to paraplegia.

Spinal-column problems have a large social significance. In Germany intervertebral-disk problems are responsible for one-fifth of all work missed because of illness and half of all early retirement requests according to the statistics of health insurance and social-security institutes. The first symptoms of this problem usually occur between the 25th and the 30th year of life. About 80 percent of the German population suffer at least once from problems connected directly or indirectly with a degenerative change in the lumbar vertebral disks.

Conservative treatment—including physical therapy, medication, and bed rest—is prescribed first. When there is no improvement and the pain become unbearable, the second option is an operation. Since the beginning of the 1960s, there has been an alternative: intra-disk injection therapy with a substance like chymopapain.

In 1964, Lyman Smith carried out the first so-called chemo-nucleolysis (spinal injection) with the plant protease chymopapain and proved its positive effect on the intervertebral-disk tissue. In

1941, Jansen and Balls isolated chymopapain from the papaya plant. This active ingredient is a proteolytic (protein-decomposing) enzyme with a molecular weight of 27,000 Dalton. It has twice the enzymatic activity of crystalline papain.

In 1956, the researcher Thomas found that giving an intravenous injection of it to young rabbits caused their ears and other cartilage tissue to become slack for a short time. The proteolytic effect of chymopapain is due to the splitting of water-attracting macromolecules in the nucleus pulposus of a disk. Chymopapain reduces the volume of the intervertebral-disk material and thereby the source of the pressure. The displaced disk tissue's pressure on the affected compressed nerve root is relaxed and sometimes there is a sudden release from the pain. The healthy tissue surrounding it remains intact.

During the 1960s and 1970s there was a real boom in chemonucleolysis with practically unanimous positive results. Up until 1975, the number of patients who were treated by this method in Germany rose to more than 16,000. At the beginning of the 1980s, a new and improved preparation with more intensive and longer-lasting enzyme activity was introduced: Chymodiactin. In a large American study ("Illinois Trial") with 1,498 patients, 85 percent of those treated had results that were considered "good" or "very good." There were also about 200,000 intra-disk injections with chymopapain by 1988, with 100,000 new patients in the USA alone.

It is possible for allergic side effects to occur in reaction to the chymopapain injection. But in comparison with other foreign proteins, it has relatively weak antigen potency. Chicken protein meets 21 times more frequently with allergic reactions and horse serum 41 times more often. However, one percent of the population of the USA has already developed antibodies against chymopapain. The increased number of incidents with chemonucleolysis is probably related to the increased use of papayas. In the USA, chymopapain or papain is found in many products such as cosmetics, toothpaste, and cleaning solutions for contact lenses or false teeth, creating the danger of sensitization.

The probability of an allergic reaction to chymopapain in chemonucleolysis lies between 0.2 and 2 percent. This figure is decreasing as a result of the allergy tests that many doctors carry out before the injection. In the Illinois study, 0.9 percent of the patients experienced an allergic reaction; two women patients, corresponding to 0.143 percent, died as a result of an allergic shock. Skin tests can almost eliminate the risk. Composite statistics in Europe of 18,925 chymopapain injections resulted only in 0.2 percent allergic reactions without death. Since H1 and H2 beta-blockers and cortisone have been given as a preventive measure before the injection in Germany, there have been no more cases of shock triggered by allergies. When local anesthetic is used, complications occur only half as frequently as they do in situations where general anesthesia is employed. Of the 1,286 patients in 44 German neurosurgical and orthopedic clinics who were injected with chymopapain, only 21 patients had allergic reactions and these were of a less severe nature.

According to many doctors, chemonucleolysis should not be used for every type of temporary backache or sciatic pain. In any case, the possibility of conservative therapy should be utilized for at least six weeks beforehand, including two weeks of strict confinement to bed.

The success rates of spinal injection lie between 70 and 95 percent. For operations, similar success quotas are reported but with ten times the number of serious complications. For this reason, many doctors think that, in the proper circumstances, chemonucleolysis should be employed as the last conservative treatment step for prolapsed disks before doing an open intervertebral disk operation. In addition, the spinal injection is less expensive; the patients remain in the hospital for shorter time periods and can go back to work or sports earlier.

A few tips:
- There are other possibilities for preventing backaches and pain in the back. Some health insurance companies contribute payment toward courses in somatic education, which teach people how to sit, stand, walk and move correctly so that the lumbar vertebral column is not subject to unnecessary stress.
- For the past five years, I have used the *Five Tibetan Rites,* a system of yoga exercises that is excellent for preventing and relieving backaches. Through these special movements, the nutrition of the intervertebral tissue is improved. My back problems due to a curved spine have disappeared as a result, but they reappear when I omit

the exercises for one day. See the book *Ancient Secret of the Fountain of Youth* by Peter Kelder for more information.
- Halima Neumann—along with Dr. John W. Ray and Dr. Kurt Koesel of Hawaii—recommends the use of unripe papayas to treat disk problems since it is assumed that papain regenerates and rebuilds cartilage. Arginine, which is split off from the simple proteins with the help of papain (also see *Papaya as a Digestive Aid* on page 91), activates the growth hormone HGH in the pineal gland. This leads to the regeneration of bone cartilage. Papaya recipes can be found in *Recipes for the Kitchen* on page 160 and under *The Papaya as a Healing Remedy* on page 167. There are a number of digestive aids based on the papaya available at natural food stores.

Homeopathic Applications for Papaya

The alkaloids in the leaves of the papaya plant—carpaine, nicotine, and carpsoid—are used in homeopathy. In their German-language homeopathic adviser on the prevention and treatment of tropical diseases, the authors Ravi Roy and Carola Lage-Roy recommend the papaya as an accompanying diet for various diseases.

Against hepatitis, the prophylactic "Hepatitis Nosode 200C" is advised. This should be accompanied by a diet of ripe papayas, eaten as fruit, and unripe papayas cooked like vegetables (with rice).

Against acute parasitic infestation, the stubborn bilharziasis (which can cause delayed damage to the bladder, liver, or intestine), a papaya diet is recommended. According to the authors, following a strict diet for three weeks should improve the chances of getting rid of the parasites. Take raw, green papaya, cut it into small pieces and cooks them with a lot of water and a little salt. Eat this papaya vegetable with rice twice a day. In addition, only drink water. After three weeks, other foods can slowly be added. When we eat food that is relatively sharply spiced, we are generally protected against worms. Eating fresh or dried papaya seeds is useful for this purpose. Eating one tablespoon of the seeds together with the sweet, ripe fruit makes their taste milder. [100]

Against typhoid, complete fasting is recommended during the fever phase. As a homeopathic remedy, one portion of "Typhoid Nosode" (Typhinum) 200C is recommended mornings and evenings. After the fever has passed, begin with ripe, juicy fruit, whereby only one type should be eaten at a time. Green, cooked bananas and papaya can be eaten with rice and yogurt.

Anyone who travels should get hold of this type of information. There are even effective "malaria nosodes" against tropical malaria that have no side effects but increase the general powers of resistance.

In the homeopathic mother tincture of the papaya, there is a silver number of 0.030 to 0.047 that indicates a low concentration of mustard oil. Advice for the application of the mother tincture (essence) or a potency of it can be found in the book *Materia Medica of Indian Drugs* by Dr. Pradas Banerjee (also see *The Papaya in the Folk Medicine of India* on page 137).

The so-called "teep" is made from young, fresh leaves. This is the starting material for the homeopathic essence. Otto Leeger's book on homeopathy recommends treating bladder problems and urinary tract pain with Papaya in a dosage of potency 4C or 5C. In the case of a moist eczema of the palm of the hand, take a dose of potency 3X or 4X.

The Papaya in Ethno-Medicine of Native Peoples

*"Every disease, every pain has its origin.
This is the price we must pay
for something done in the past
or even in the future."*

(Rolling Thunder, medicine man from the Cherokee tribe)

*"Papaya is the gift of the gods
for people with a sad stomach."*

(Indian saying)

Many old medicinal-herb recipes of native peoples are being re-discovered; books and seminars about ethno-medicine are in demand. This scientific branch developed about 20 years ago through the mutual efforts of ethnologists, biologists, and physicians. Ethno-physicians study the way diseases are treated and healed by spending years living with the tribes. Their aim is to research the way native peoples who live close to nature practice healing and, as far as possible, to integrate this knowledge to our Western cultures.

Ethno-medicine informs us of the ancient knowledge regarding the healing powers of plants and preserves this knowledge for us so that it can be put to use. If you would like to know more about this group, you can to write the "AGEM", an alliance of about 500 scientists, ethnologists, physicians, psychologists, and midwives; they organize lectures and publish books about the knowledge they have accumulated in their long research travels.

The compiled examples illustrate how the papaya has been used for centuries as a medicinal plant. These may serve as an inspiration for healing practitioners, physicians, manufacturers of natural healing remedies, and laypeople who want to take greater advantage of the exceptional medicinal properties of this tropical fruit.

Three of four plant ingredients in our medications have been derived from the knowledge of the tropical rain forest Indians and other "guards of the forests." "Indigenous" people originally cultivated a large number of useful plants, upon which the world's nutrition is based today. Scientists assume that the Indian forest tribes have developed more than 90 percent of all human knowledge about the use of animal and plant species.

The Organization ARA (Society for the Protection of the Rain Forest and Species) supports the Indian people in their fight to keep their homelands. A health center in the state of Rondonia, Brazil is attempting to compile the existing traditional knowledge of the individual tribes so that it can be preserved and put to use. ARA also supports projects in Costa Rica and Vietnam, negotiates with politicians worldwide, and spreads information about the possibilities of preserving the forests with their biological potential and protecting the people living in them in their brochures, books (also for children), lectures, and seminars. Every dollar contributed is multiplied by five through the support of public funding so that it is optimally invested for the actual aim.

In an essay by Chung-Shih Tang, there is an—incomplete—survey on the "Use of Papaya in Folk Medicine" in "Tropical Foods, vol. 1", page 56. I am in contact with Professor Tang, and we will attempt to compile a more complete list of "patient information for natural healing".

The Papaya in Native Central and South American Plant Therapy

The tropical papaya was originally a Central American plant and comes from southern Mexico and Costa Rica. It is an old Indian cult plant. The Indians of Central and South America use the papaya to heal virtually everything and call it the "tree of health." Papaya trees are still planted for their pleasant-tasting fruit and the outstanding medicinal properties of the entire plant.

The papaya fruit was already used by the Mayas for **constipation**, a "sluggish liver," and **digestive problems**, as well as high blood pressure and intestinal parasites. Diego de Landa, the first Bishop of Yucatan, noted the digestive properties of the papaya at the beginning of the 16th century. Regarding the medicinal usage by the Mayas, the colonial text *Libro de Judio* says: "The virtues of this plant are wonderful. One eats the fruit to stimulate digestion and the gallbladder; the juice normalizes the activity of the stomach and the gallbladder and the function of the liver. The milk juice contained in the bark and green fruit heals diarrhea immediately. It is also good for treating asthma and expelling of worms. The seeds, pulverized and drunk, expel tapeworm."[101] According to an old Mayan text, the roots were also used as a remedy: "The fire, that burns in men (...) take for this (...) the root of the Papaya (...) grind it and smear it on the skin; this will heal it."[102]

The fruit and the pulverized seeds are still applied to infected wounds and injuries by the Indians today. Even the crushed pulp of the fruit is an excellent **wound remedy**, which is said to heal the most difficult injuries quickly. The Mexican Indians mix dried papaya seeds (one tablespoon) with a cup of water and pumpkinseeds in the sun (alternative: oven at low temperature) and apply the thickened paste to sprains, bruises, contusions, and **small injuries.**

The milky juice, which flows out of the unripe fruit when it is scratched, is used for **skin rashes and burns**. If a burn is treated with the juice immediately, no blisters form and the pain disappears immediately.

Caution: Be careful not to get this liquid in your eyes because it may cause impaired vision.

The Indians also use the latex juice of the unripe papaya with success for **warts**. The juice that comes out when the stem is scratched is used for dissolving **corns on the feet**. Extracts from the roots are used to treat **arthritic pain**. The cooked root is a component of a recipe against **genital diseases**. Papaya juice is also used as a universal antidote for **animal bites**. Rubbing the afflicted spot with very ripe or even rotten fruit can reduce redness and irritation caused by corals.

On his travels, Alfred Vogel observed that the natives of South America put pieces of papaya leaves the size of half-dollars in their mouths and chewed them several times a day in order to protect themselves from **infectious diseases** and epidemics. Papaya regener-

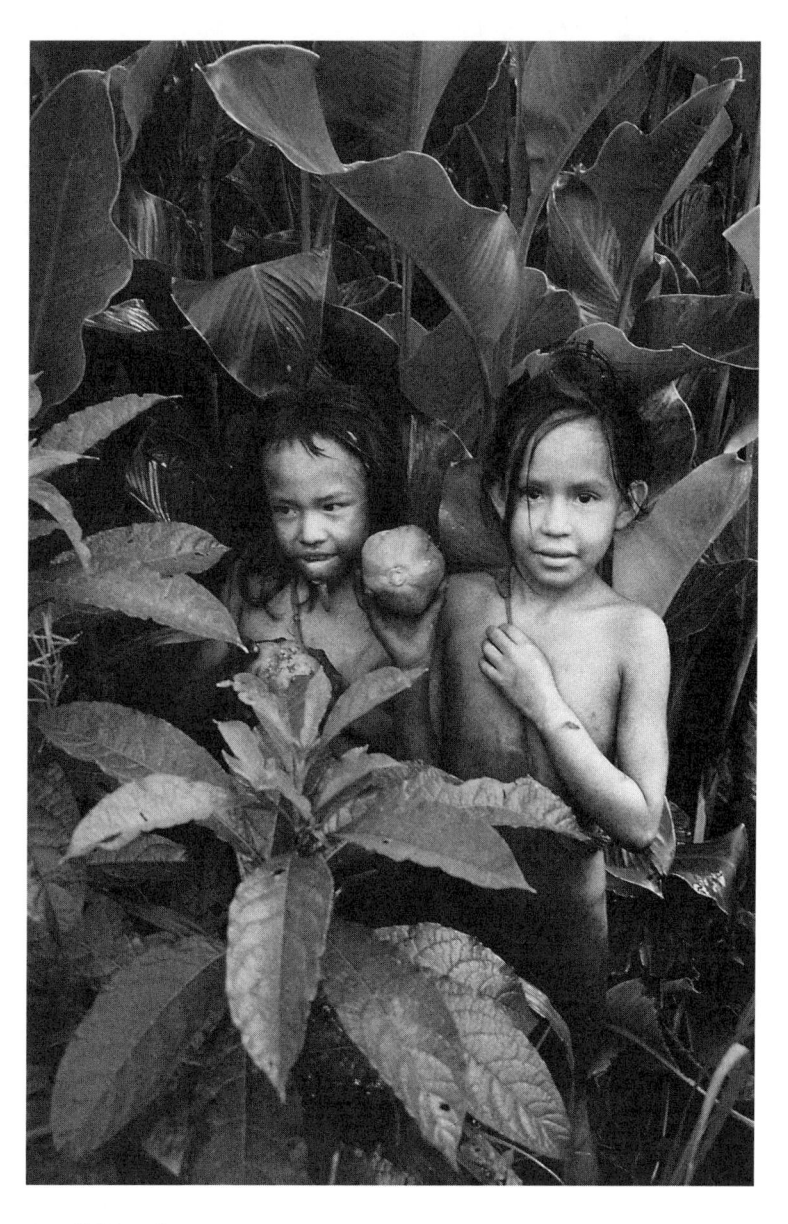

Brazil, Mato Grosso:
Girls from the Nambi Cuara tribe with green papaya

ates the intestinal flora and has an antibacterial effect; for this reason, the Indian medicine men use them for **diarrhea** (raw with some salt). If there are no papayas at hand, eat pieces of pineapple mixed with chili pods (strongly salted).

The Indians get rid of amebas and **worms** by chewing the leaves or seeds of the papaya fruit. A tea made from leaves and seeds is also taken for worms. The Indians use tea from dried leaves, which contain carpaine, for **high blood pressure and heart problems**. The juice from the unripe fruit is still used today for **high blood pressure** in Guyana and a few of the Caribbean islands.

Bronchitis is considered to be an "arrow disease." Recipes using papaya leaves and pumpkinseeds come from Central America. The leaves are cooked with half a quart of water and then filtered. Sip this brew hot twice a day, upon rising and before going to bed. Pumpkinseeds are cooked with some salt and one tablespoon of them is taken several times a day.

The Indians of Central and South America use the root of the papaya plant against **kidney and bladder problems**. The ripe fruit is eaten for **beriberi** and the milk juice used to curdle milk.

R. E. Schultes reports in his book *The Healing Forest, Medical and Toxic Plants of the Northwest Amazonia* that the Indian tribe Tikunas uses the papaya to induce **miscarriages**. For this purpose, the Tikuna women eat the grated, unripe fruit together with two to six aspirins. The embryo is then expelled two days after taking this remedy. There is also information on the use of the papaya as an abortive and a contraceptive in India and Papua-New Guinea (see section on Contraceptives in the A-Z section). In Polynesia, women are reported to chew 25 seeds a day in order to prevent conception (no guarantee!). For this reason, seeds of the ripe fruit and pulp of the unripe fruit should not be consumed in larger quantities during pregnancy!

In Central and South America, the papaya has also been used to treat cancer for centuries. The author Gerhard Leibold has therefore called these Indians the "founders of enzyme therapy against cancer". They apparently were instinctively aware that papaya is among the most important plant enzyme carriers. Hundreds of years later, Dr. Wolf and Dr. Christian identified the immune substance that prevents cancer growth in healthy beings and can destroy cancer cells to be the protein-splitting enzyme.

The natives of South America also use tea from papaya blossoms for **fever, asthma,** and **bronchitis.** The Indians view asthma as a "wind infection." In general, the original inhabitants of Central and South America value the papaya as a delicacy that not only tastes good but is also beneficial for health. They eat a piece of the fruit after almost every meal in order to digest heavy foods more easily. They know that the papaya relieves nausea after indulging in fatty foods or alcohol.

The Papaya in the Folk Medicine of India

It probably isn't true that the papaya first came to China and India after the discovery of America, as it says in many books. There were already references to it in ancient Chinese history books. In India, the use of *Carica papaya* is extraordinarily popular. The entire plant is used. The milk juice is employed against all kinds of **skin diseases** in India. If **burns** are immediately rubbed with it, no blisters form.

The latex juice is used to remove **freckles, senile speckles, and skin blotches** caused by sunshine. For Diphtheria, they paint the throat with the papaya's milk juice. The latex, which contains papain, is also applied to **warts** in India. If this doesn't work, they bind a piece of the bark over the wart for 24 hours, after which it usually disappears. For **rickets,** they rub the lower extremities with an alcoholic root extract of the papaya.

For **arthritic pain,** the following oil is used: fill a wine bottle half full with pieces of papaya root, add one tablespoon of cooking salt and two spoons of eucalyptus oil. Then fill the bottle with a spirit such as brandy and place the tightly closed bottle in the sun for ten days. The painful area is then rubbed with this papaya oil every evening. It is also used for **muscle tension, muscle weakness,** and muscle paralysis after a **stroke.**

The blossoms of the papaya are steamed in milk and butter to **stimulate the appetite** and given especially to weak, listless children to eat. The desire to eat is also supposedly stimulated by a mixture of raw, young leaves pounded with salt and mixed with water. It is mainly given to pale, skinny children.

The ripe fruit is generally eaten for **stomach problems, digestive disorders,** and **rectal inflammation**. It supports digestion and is good for the pancreas. In addition, raw papaya induces contractions of muscle fibers of the stomach and promotes a light and distinct **menstrual flow.**

The milk juice of the papaya is taken mixed 1:1 with water in a liquor glass to dispel pinworms, ascarids, and other **intestinal parasites**; it is also used against abdominal colic and secretion of mucus from the intestine. In order to get rid of worms, eucalyptus oil is taken the next day to expel them.

Here is another recipe for pinworms: cook the roots together with garlic in one cup of water until half of it has evaporated and the mixture is thick. Half of this amount is taken twice a day with milk. Children should eat very little food during this treatment; probably because this facilitates the breakdown of proteins by the papain (see also *Papaya Gets Rid of Worms* on pages 124 ff).

The young leaves cooked as vegetables have a choleretic (gall-stimulating) effect. In addition, the leaves are said to generally reduce fever and cleanse the liver. Raw papaya is also good for people with **liver problems**. Young papaya leaves are eaten to fight **malaria** and given to young children with irregular bowel movements. The juice from the raw leaves helps women with **vaginal discharge**: the young leaves are extracted in salt water after soaking for fifteen days. When the bark is cooked, the result is an infusion with which **gout in the foot** is healed in India. The recommendation for **syphilis** is drinking liquor-glass portions of this infusion.

For fever connected with **colds and flu,** rub an infusion of the finely pounded seeds mixed with vinegar onto the skin. This is said to increase perspiration. In India, cows are fed green papaya leaves in order to improve their digestion. Descriptions of the papaya in the folk medicine of India can also be found in the book "Materia Medica of Indian Drugs" by Dr. Prasad Banerjee (see *Bibliography*).

The Papaya in Ayurveda— India's Ancient Method of Healing and Way of Life

Ayurveda means "teaching of a (long) life." Ether, air, fire, water, and earth are the five basic elements, manifesting themselves in the human body as the basic principles or humors of the body called the "three doshas" or "tridoshas." They regulate the formation, preservation, and destruction of the body tissue and the elimination of waste products. In addition, they are also responsible for psychological phenomena such as feelings ranging from love to anger.

The principal of air and ether manifests itself in the body as Vata; the elements of fire and water make themselves apparent as Pitta; and the elements of earth and water appear as the bodily fluids, which are called Kapha. According to Ayurvedic teachings, a balanced condition among the three doshas is the basic prerequisite for physical and mental health. "A basic principle of healing in Ayurveda, holds that one can create balance in the internal forces working in the individual by altering diet and habits or living to counteract changes in his internal environment."[103]

The papaya is recommended to balance the constitutional basic types of Vata and Pitta in Ayurveda. It creates the energy called "virja" (hot energy) in the body and thereby kindles "agni," the digestive fire. In turn, toxins are burned by better digestion.

A person who has an excess of Vata, like me, and eats lots of papayas will feel more grounded, more content, and more balanced emotionally since the papaya increases the Pitta. Someone with a Vata constitution—who basically corresponds with the slender, easily exhausted, and nervous "movement" disposition—undoubtedly needs to eat many sweet fruits such as bananas, grapes, and cherries. Kapha people are generally healthy and balanced. Physically and mentally, they move slowly and have a tendency toward being overweight. If the Kapha disposition is too pronounced, they tend toward apprehension, envy, and a greed for possessions. Pitta people cannot bear sunshine, heat, or hard physical work very well. They are generally ambitious in terms of leadership roles and tend emotionally toward hate, anger, and jealousy. Papaya reduces the gallbladder activity (typical of Pitta-oriented people) and helps against the health disorders that are caused by an excess of Pitta.

As in the teachings of Natural Hygiene (compare especially with *Cancer—Causes and Alternatives* on pages 95 ff), the Ayurvedic system sees "ama"—waste deposits or toxemia—as responsible for all illness. However, in this health system toxins do not occur just because of incompatible foods that cannot be digested well together, eating too quickly or irregularly, but also through emotional factors. Similar to Buddhism, Ayurveda teaches that we can release all of our negative feelings through consciousness.

In Indian Ayurveda, the papaya *(Papitá* in Hindi) is prescribed for disturbances of the gastro-intestinal secretion (we would probably call this "enzyme deficiency"), **infections of the pancreas**, intestinal worms, **skin diseases,** and **hardening of the liver.** In addition, it is prescribed for **dyspepsia** associated with decompensated heart disease since papaya contains carpaine, which works similarly to digitalis. The pulp is eaten when the spleen is enlarged, something that frequently occurs in the case of cancer. In Ayurveda, hot papaya is a good remedy for strengthening the liver function. In addition, the papaya supports urine excretion and helps to release a Vata excess of gases in the intestine more easily (flatulence).

In the Ayurvedic teaching, the papaya is recommended only against **constipation** but not when there is diarrhea. According to the three "gunas," "sattva" is light, clarity, and knowledge; rajas is inspiration, activity, and pain; tamas is doubt, darkness, and force. Sattva, which has the highest vibrations, allows us to become light and full of energy, to experience bliss and joy, and to bring our soul into a state of harmony. In order to develop more sattva, a diet consisting only of sweet fruits is ideal. Freshly squeezed fruit juices from sweet, ripe fruits like the papaya are considered the purest sattvic foods (see *Papaya Juice—a Health Cocktail* on pages 59 ff). Papaya has a high glycemic index, which means that it is quickly metabolized. Please keep this in mind if you have hypoglycemia (also see *Enter the Zone: A Dietary Road Map to Lose Weight Permanently* by Berry Sears and Bill Lawren).

The Papaya in Chinese Medicine

The papaya was described in the Chinese medical plant book *Bencao gangmu* from the 16th century. It was written between 1552 and 1578. In other ancient Chinese medicinal plant books, the papaya is designated as the "fruit of a long life" because it has the power to make everything digestible that cannot be digested. The Chinese call the papaya *fanmugua,* whereby *fan* means foreign and indicates that the fruit was introduced from a foreign land, probably through the Philippines.

Traditionally, the papaya is used in China to treat **digestive disturbances, constipation, stomachaches, urinary complaints, rheumatism, and ulcers.** The fruit is either eaten raw or boiled in water and this decoction is drunk. Primarily the unripe, green papaya is used against digestive complaints and stomachaches; for dysentery, urinary complaints, and constipation, the ripe fruit is used.

When they breastfeed, Cantonese women eat green papaya together with meat to stimulate the flow of milk. For this purpose, they cook a small green half-pound papaya and 2 ounces of lean pork gently in 2 quarts of water for one hour until only a pint of thick fluid is left. The nursing woman then drinks the milky broth and eats as much of the papaya and meat as possible. The soup should be eaten for a number of days.

For **skin sores** and **inflammations**, the papaya leaves are mashed and used to
 cover the afflicted spots. Two to three pieces of the ripe papaya are eaten in cases of **constipation** (but diarrhea is the result when too much is eaten).

The Papaya in Voodoo Medicine

Voodoo is practiced in larger parts of black Africa and in Caribbean countries like Haiti. In his German-language book on voodoo medicine, Uwe Karsten describes a recipe for using the papaya as a poultice for **bruises, warts,** and **ringworm:** the ingredients are a papaya leaf, a quarter teaspoon of pork fat, and a bandage. The leaf is washed thoroughly, removing all foreign material. Then it is grated, mixed with the fat, and placed on the skin. After this, it is carefully covered with a bandage. This procedure should be repeated for four to five days.

The Papaya in the Folk Medicine of Nigeria, Ghana, and Iboland

In Nigeria, people smoke the dried leaves of the papaya when they have breathing difficulties such as **coughs, asthma, and bronchitis** in order to soothe the upper respiratory tract. Researchers have found four substances in alcohol extracts of the papaya leaves: carpaine, pseudocarpaine, nicotine, and an additional, as yet unidentified alkaloid. Smoking just one or two cigarettes made of papaya leaves also results in an acceleration of the brain waves, relaxation of the muscles, and a clear increase in the concentration of the growth hormone, the antiduretic hormone, and glycerin in the blood plasma.

Corresponding experiments with rats verify that the papaya leaves have a relaxing effect on the central nervous system and reduce the sensation of pain. In the light of these observations, it would be valuable to study how the strong sedative effects of papaya leaves and their extracts could be used in surgery, to protect epileptics from seizures, and in electrotherapy.

Moreover, in northern Nigeria a cold-water extract is made from the fruit in order to control and relax people who are mentally overexcited and "flipping out." The mashed leaves and seeds are eaten against **worms** and **fever**.

In Iboland (southeastern Nigeria) and Ghana, an extract of the dried leaves is used for **stomach and digestive problems**. In Ghana, the papaya is also given against **jaundice, ringworm, and intestinal parasites**, as well as against **fever, beriberi,** and **amebic dysentery**. The root is used for kidney and bladder disorders and **hemorrhoids**.

In Zimbabwe, the medicine men use the papaya for babies whose fontanel is depressed. They use grated roots mixed with gruel. As an alternative, papaya roots are cooked with bananas or lemon tree roots and given as an infusion.

The Papaya as a Healing Plant of the Kahunas, Hawaii

The *Kahunas-La'au-Lapa'au* in Hawaii have also applied papayas, and they still use them today. Kahuna originally meant "high priest" or "guardian of the secrets." The modern translation would be "master of healing herbs" and would correspond to our doctor's degree.

In Hawaiian, the papaya is called *mikana*. It is used for the following health disorders:

1. **Cancer** in the early stage: Eat papaya seeds several times a day.

2. **Digestive problems**: Papaya seeds are eaten or dried and grated and used on food instead of pepper.

3. **Wounds, cuts, open areas**: To remove poisons, the bottoms side (shade side) of the Lau-Kahi leaf (broad-leafed plantain, Latin: *Plantago major L.*), is laid on the wound. In order to heal, the upper side (sun side) is laid over it. Then the milk juice of the papaya with the active ingredient papain is spread over it.

According to Dietrich Kempski, from whom I have this information, worm illnesses occurred very rarely in Hawaii. If they did occur, the ripe, soft, pale nonI fruit (Indian mulberry, *Morinda citrifolia L*) was dried in the sun and eaten like a fruit. There was no indication in his work of the papaya's use in curing worm infestation.

I was fortunate that a *kahuna pule,* who heals with the power of prayer and has been also healing with the power of the papaya for many years now, also sent me a long report. She assists a kahuna in Kihei on Maui.

In order to induce **birth**, the woman drinks this papaya beverage: seven peanut shells, a papaya leaf, and seven pistachios. Cover everything with boiling water and let it brew for twenty minutes. If nothing happens, mix a raw egg white with papaya juice and drink one hour later.

Here is the kahuna recipe for **intestinal parasites**: Mix papaya juice with an equal proportion of honey and drink it in hot coffee. Half an hour later, take one full tablespoon of castor oil. Astara Kim Hill

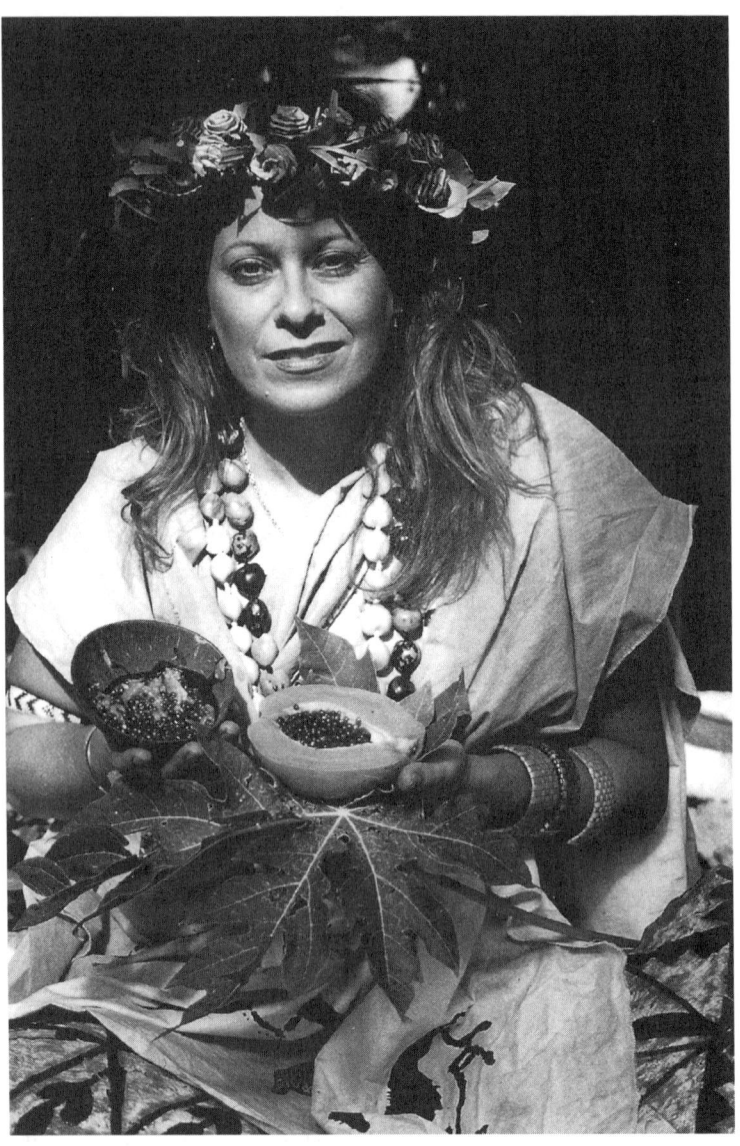

Native Havaiian (Astara Kim Hill) with papaya

writes that papaya juice is the most effective remedy against worms that the kahunas know. In order to get rid of worms quickly, one can go to a papaya tree and scratch the green fruit in several places; collect the milk juice and drink slowly. To counteract weight loss following parasite infestation, cut the papaya root into small pieces, cook it with a little water, and drink this four times a day between meals. Children who have worms are given between 2/3 and 1 ounce of cabbage juice and papaya juice, followed by a slice of fresh pineapple.

In order to prevent **cancer**, the kahunas from Hawaii eat dates (which contain much magnesium), raw onions or garlic, and papaya seeds twice a month (or more frequently). When cancer patients have pain, they are given juice from papayas and strawberries with natural raw sugar or sugar juice. For leukemia, the patient takes a drink composed of 5 grams of calendula and 5 grams of daisies in a quart of milk, boiled with some green papaya.

For **asthma attacks,** take three leaves of aloe vera and make a juice of their pulp. Mix this with three teaspoons of strong coffee. When the person has calmed down, he or she should eat a slice of ripe papaya. Otherwise, asthmatics should drink papaya juice and smell the fragrance of the belladonna flower (do not eat, poisonous!). An alternative: Mix papaya leaves and almond leaves, make a tea of them, and eat three to five slices of papaya with it.

Patients with **rheumatism** can bathe in water with leaves of cherimoya, lemon, papaya, and belladonna plants added to it. Allow the leaves to steep in the hot water and then take a bath in the water.

The following drink is recommended against **syphilis**: Seeds from half of a papaya are put in warm water. Drink this water until the illness is gone.

To heal **skin sores,** boil a papaya leaf in castor oil and pork fat. This is applied as a compress for one to three hours.

For **bladder infections,** the papaya roots are boiled and the water mixed with fresh parsley juice. This liquid is taken before meals. If available, young coconuts can be eaten with it.

For **wounds and cuts,** apply the milk juice of the papaya and cover this area with a papaya leaf.

A tea against **bronchitis** can be made from papaya flowers by pouring boiling water over the flowers and drinking the decoction. Another possibility is eating papaya three times a day together with a hibiscus flower.

For a **lymph gland infection:** Boil the leaves of the papaya and pour the resulting tea into a prepared warm bath. Two cups of stone salt can be added to it in order to extract toxins from the lymph system. Rub the leaves into the lymph region (with a wet towel soaked in the leaf decoction). Everything should be as hot as tolerable.

For **constipation**, drink three slices of papaya dissolved in half a glass of warm water with one teaspoon of stone salt or sea salt.

Against **toothaches**, make a paste of fresh papaya roots and smear it on the teeth and gums.

For **diarrhea**, grate green papayas, pour water over them, and allow them to sit for a few minutes. Then sieve and take three times a day with a teaspoon of juice from green or ripe papayas. This recipe is also good for children.

For **stomachache**, drink a decoction made of the small masculine flowers and water for seven days.

For **muscle pain**, pulverize one papaya leaf, mix it with castor oil, apply this mixture around the area, and place a warm towel over it. Such warm compresses can also be placed on the stomach for stomach complaints.

The same mixture can be enriched with four noni leaves and used on the breasts as a compress for **breast cancer** (three to four hours at a time for at least five days).

Note: Dried, fermented papaya leaves used to make teas, compresses, etc. can be obtained from the Firm Papaya Force. See *Resources* on page 207.

There are additional recipes that I cannot include for reasons of space. Astara concludes "People should feel the spirit of the mikana plant, regardless of where it grows in the world, and ask the plant if it wants to help before using it." Furthermore, if we treat others, we should be aware of our motivation for ourselves and for the patient at all stages of the treatment.

The Papaya as a Healing Plant of the Aborigines

Since the appearance of the article about papaya as "the cancer-healing plant of the Aborigines" by Ruediger Schlegel in the German magazine "Bio" (No. 1/1997), this plant has been discussed as a healing remedy in German-speaking areas. Many naturopathically oriented people use it for the prevention and healing of cancer.

In the above-mentioned article, the story is told of the patient June Benett from Pottsville Beach, Australia, who was diagnosed by the doctors as having **lung cancer**. However, she didn't want to accept the death sentence and researched for naturopathic alternatives. By drinking papaya tea (a type of ancient secret Aborigine recipe) for three months, a remarkable improvement in her condition became apparent. The **bone cancer**, which developed after three years, was also reported to have been healed by the papaya tea.

According to Schlegel, one can cook the skin of the unripe fruit as an alternative to the tea from papaya leaves. The cancer researcher Dr. Antoine Palade is reported to have said in an interview with the Australian *Sunday Mail* of April 9, 1995 that he had successfully treated people and animals with a papaya skin tincture against **skin cancer**.

In his books *Kombucha: The Miracle Fungus* and *Papaya—The Medicine Tree*, Harald Tietze describes the tea recipe of the Aborigines against cancer: Wash seven medium-sized papaya leaves that are not too old and not too young, and dry them. Then cut them finely like

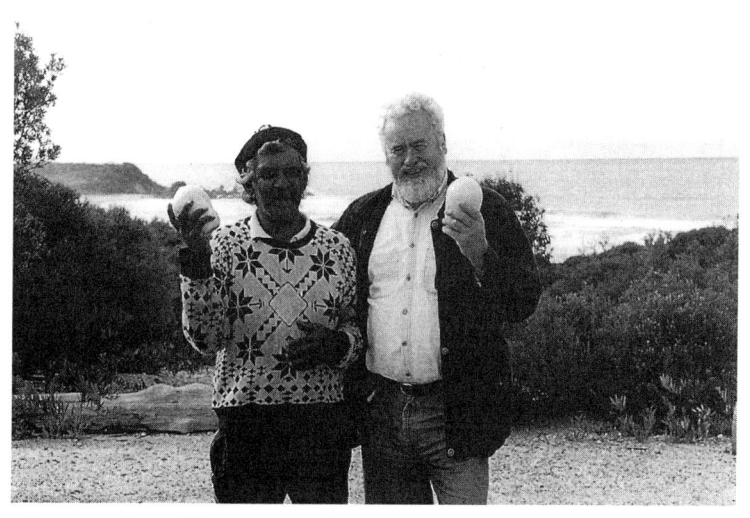

Aborigin and Harald Tietze

white cabbage and boil in two quarts of water until just one quart of the fluid is left. Filter the fluid and fill into glass containers. This can be kept in the refrigerator for three to four days, but should be discarded when it becomes cloudy in color. Every day, drink 1/4 cup three times. This decoction can also be mixed with other juices.

If you don't live in the USA, Germany, Australia or tropic regions and cannot get papaya leaves, you can also use a half-green, unripe papaya with its seeds and skin. Either make a tea according to the above recipe (I have tried it and found it to be very bitter) or cut into small pieces in a mixer together with other fruit. According to Harald Tietze, the fresh fruit has the same healing power as the available preparations and teas.

However, Dr. Wolf-Dieter Storl, a well-known ethno-physician and book author wrote me in a letter dated May 20, 1997: "The papaya has not been established very long in Australia, and I very much doubt that the plant has been a traditional healing plant of the Australian natives. It is possible that an Aborigine healer used the plant as a cancer remedy, but I doubt this since generally foreign plants don't play a role in the traditional totemistic rituals." At the totem festivals, the spirit beings in plants and animals are honored. On this occasion, plants are the center of attention and are eaten in order to support their reproduction and growth.

Harald Tietze conceded that it could not be an "ancient or traditional healing plant of the Aborigines." He wrote the following to me in his fax of July 1, 1997: "During the last decades there have been individual reports of Aborigines giving white Australians recipes for using the papaya against various illnesses, especially against cancer. These reports about a successful treatment with papaya became very popular, leading to the erroneous assumption that it is a traditional Aboriginal healing plant. Yet, it is still true that the papaya is a healing plant used by the Aborigines, a fact that is recognized not only in other Western countries but also in Australia. (...) The papaya is very much respected by the Aborigines not only as a healing plant, but also as a fruit to maintain health."

Apparently, the Aborigines often cannot explain the healing effect of plants. When people ask "why?" the answer is "that's just how it is." For more logically oriented people, such an answer is not very satisfying. Aborigines, who work in mines, are said to intuitively foresee mine accidents and simply disappear in the bush before the event. Perhaps they school their **intuition** with papaya: They use the sweetly fragrant papaya blossoms in order to contact their "higher self."

There is more information about how the Aborigines use the healing power of the papaya in Harald Tietze's informative and inspiring book *Papaya (Pawpaw), The Medicine Tree*.

The Papaya in Beauty Care

Enzymes and vitamins have also been used in the field of cosmetics for some time. Particularly the research areas of "skin aging" and "wrinkle formation" have been intensively occupied with the theme of enzymes for a number of years. Enzymes bring nutrients to the skin cells and eliminate toxins and waste substances from the organism through the skin pores. We have more than 100 perspiration glands in a single square centimeter of skin! Perspiring is not only necessary for life, but also makes a person beautiful. Ideal for this purpose are sports, sauna visits, or work in the garden. The skin has an important mission to fulfill in our immune system, which can be effectively supported by a diet and cosmetics rich in enzymes and vitamins (coenzymes that need the enzymes for their work).

Today we primarily find "free-radical catchers" such as vitamin E and C, beta carotene, and selenium in cosmetic products. Anticellulite creams with enzymes are also available. Some skin-care lines for mature skin contain the so-called SOD enzyme, superoxide dismutase, that inhibit the premature formation of wrinkles and premature aging of the skin by protecting it against damaging free radicals, toxins from the environment, and UV radiation. There is a great future for enzymes in cosmetics since they strengthen the defense mechanisms of the skin and protect us from many damaging environmental influences. In addition, they are capable of protecting and repairing elastic fibers and collagen fibers. This means that they can protect against wrinkling and even "smooth out" wrinkles that already exist from inside.

As expected, the enzyme-rich papaya is also used for beauty purposes. There are entire cosmetic lines based on the papaya, with products for cleaning, smoothing, and regenerating the skin. Because of the enzymes, the skin cells that have died are removed and digested. After a treatment with papaya enzymes, the complexion appears youthful, taut, and fresh.

In 1972, Chester French described various cosmetic products with a papaya basis in his book *Papaya—The Melon of Health*. The papaya face cream *Payacado Cream*, the production of which already began in 1937, is described here as an excellent cleansing agent for the skin. It makes the skin soft and supple, even removing the freckles that develop from staying in the sun too long. This ointment, a mixture of papain and avocado oil, supposedly sells well even without advertising. Another cream, *Maya-Papaya* was developed in 1970 and enjoys great popularity as a moisturizing and cleansing cream for the skin.

An entire line, the Green Papaya Enzyme Products, was developed by Beauty Naturally (P.O. Box 4905, Burlingame, CA 94011) on the basis of papain from the green papaya: *Skin Zyme* (enzyme mask), *Clean Zyme* (enzyme cleansing cream), *Green Papaya Enzyme Cleanser* (face cleans cream), and Green *Magic Grains* (a powder from the green papaya). The development of this line, from which the first two products have been successfully offered since 1987, was celebrated by the manufacturer as "one of the greatest breakthroughs in skin care of all time."

As we get older, the skin's regenerative power is reduced: The layer of dead skin cells becomes thicker and harder, fine lines and then deep folds develop. Through the active papaya enzyme papain in these products, the dead skin layers are softened and dissolved while healthy skin is not attacked. In addition, the growth of new skin cells is stimulated and the tissue is tightened. The products are even compatible with sensitive skin (I have tried them myself).

There are other outstanding cosmetic products on the basis of papaya. Among them is a fragrant, honey-yellow shower lotion called Source Papaya Body Wash. The firm donates ten percent of the profits for the preservation of rain forests. The firm Shaman with its *Papaya & Peppermint Extra Body Shampoo* for fine and thin hair has a similar approach: Five percent of its earnings are used for environmental purposes. This shampoo makes hair soft and shiny.

I have had excellent experiences with a *Fresh Papaya Enzyme Peel* mask. It makes the skin wonderfully smooth and rosy. The mask is also able to repair sun damage, senile speckles, and discoloration. It is also applicable to sensitive skin, but an allergy test should be done first because some people are allergic to papain.

The *Elle Beauty* website has an article on "Miami, Relaxing with Style" in which the Delano Hotel in Miami Beach, Florida offers a 90-minute "Deluxe Aroma Facial" consisting of a neck, head, and hand massage with papaya enzymes and essential oils that makes the skin supple. Since the hotel opened in 1995, such Hollywood personalities like Donna Karan and Madonna have praised the $75 treatment. The magazine *Elle* gave the "Deluxe Aroma Facial" therapy a "Beauty Oscar."

In German-speaking countries, there are few cosmetics based on papayas, except for those distributed by the firm Papaya Vera. In the Feb. 26, 1997 issue, the German women's magazine *Für Sie* published an article explaining how to make a papaya mask:

"An exotic mask for a smooth complexion: Mash the fruit pulp of a papaya with a fork and stir in 1—2 teaspoons of cream to make a smooth paste. Apply to a clean face. Let it take effect for 30 minutes, then wash off." I have tried the recipe successfully using avocado instead of cream.

In response to my question about papaya products, the magazine editor wrote: "As far as we know, there is not yet a cosmetic product in Germany using papaya extract. Unfortunately, you must use the *fruit pure* for now. A beauty treatment from within is also good: Have a fruit day during which you eat only pineapple and papaya. It works like a major cleansing of the body." The same idea is found in a book about enzymes as active components for women: If you want to pamper your skin, don't just use cosmetics containing enzymes, but take enzymes in tablet form as well!"[104]

Eating fresh fruit is naturally just as good. The seeds of the ripe papaya and the pulp of the less-than-ripe fruit in particular contain a great deal of papain. Here is a recipe for a massage oil, which also helps against muscle tension, that has been handed down in India: "Fill a wine bottle to the halfway point with little pieces of the Carica papaya root, add a tablespoon of table salt and two spoons of eucalyptus-alba oil, and then fill the bottle with brandy. Close it tightly and leave it in the sun for ten days. Before you go to sleep at night, rub it onto the painful areas. This oil is also good for muscle weakness, particularly for rubbing into women's muscles after childbirth and as a massage oil in general."[105]

If you can get half-ripe or green papayas, you can also cut the fruit and rub your face with white latex juice the way the beautiful South Sea women did a century ago in order to cleanse and clarify the skin. For an intensive treatment (also against freckles, warts, and pimples), dry the seeds of the ripe papaya and apply together with avocado as paste. This mask contains a great deal of papain and works well. Since it looks terrible, choose a time when the postman won't be ringing the doorbell!

In Australia, there is an ointment (made by Kneipp Cure, Dapto) that works very well for sunburn. Since the ozone hole is growing and sun radiation is expected to increase, there will certainly be a market for such a plant product in the future.

In conclusion, here are a few recipes that you can make yourself:

FACIAL MASK FOR FRESH, SMOOTH SKIN
1/3 papaya
1 teaspoon honey
1 egg yoke
1 avocado
1 teaspoon olive oil
Mix all the ingredients and apply the mask to the cleansed skin. Let it take affect for about 15 minutes. Carefully wash off with warm water.

RELAXING PAPAYA BATH ADDITIVE
quart of papaya juice or tea (from dried leaves or fruit peels) or quart lemon-balm or chamomile tea

3 drops of lavender oil
Fill the bathtub with water first, and then add the mixture.
REFRESHING PAPAYA BATH ADDITIVE
1/4 quart papaya juice or tea (from dried leaves or fruit peel)
3 drops each of lemon oil, orange oil, and neruli oil
You will feel energetic and be in a good mood after this bath. It should last about 20 minutes.

PAPAYA OIL
For this oil, cut the skin of one papaya into small pieces and put them in a pot (not made of aluminum since papain attacks aluminum). Add olive or sunflower oil until everything is covered well and boil gently for 5 minutes. Put it in a cool place for two days. Then press it through a cloth and pour it into a bottle. You can rub the face and body with this oil. It has a refreshing effect and nourishes the skin. If you wish, you can mix it with calendula or almond oil.
It can also be used as a massage oil for the stomach when you are constipated, suffer from flatulence, and have any other digestive disturbances. A massage with papaya oil also helps against coughs and bronchitis, as well as heart problems caused by nervousness.

PAPAYA VINEGAR (FOR SALAD AND BATHS)
Cut the fruit skin, the entire fruit, or the papaya leaves (dry or fresh) into thin slices. Then pour this into a preserve jar until it is two-thirds full and add apple-cider vinegar.
This papaya vinegar will keep for a long time. If you use it as a bath additive, your skin will become smooth and taut. In addition, it is good against infections. Dandruff disappears when the hair is rinsed a number of times with papaya vinegar.

Papaya John—A Life for Papayas

"Papaya—that's my mission!"
(John McCollum alias Papaya John)

In Paia, a sleepy wind-surfing spot on the Hawaiian Island of Maui, there is a small store called Papaya John's. It has only papaya products. What convinced John McCollum, the owner, to spend his whole life spreading the "Papaya Gospel" of the healing qualities of this "tropical wonder fruit"?

Even when John surfs, he uses the opportunity to advertise for papayas: A huge papaya is painted on his surfboard. He sees himself as the successor of Dr. Koesel, a German who became extremely ill in the Caribbean during the 1930s. He was cared for by native nurses and treated exclusively with papaya. In an unbelievably short time, he was completely healthy again. Consequently, Dr. Koesel experimented with the papaya and, together with Dr. Ray (who now lives in Australia), healed many people with the juice of the green fruit. One of these individuals was the German Halima Neumann, who had cancer of the urinary tract (see *Papain in Enzyme Therapy against Cancer* on page 103 ff).

In the 1970s, John McCollum, who was a hippie at that time, met Dr. Koesel and knew immediately: "This meeting is magical, I am karmically connected to this old man." He decided to help Dr. Koesel and to work for him. In return, Dr. Koesel initiated him into the health secrets of the papaya. John is especially enthusiastic about its effects as a digestive aid: "When you eat a piece of my dried papaya bar with a meal, the nutrients are absorbed better, you have more energy, and you free your body of waste materials."

In 1990, when Dr. Koesel died one week before his 90th birthday, things were clear for John McCollum: "I have made an agreement with God and Dr. Koesel. I believe in what the papaya can do and it's my task to make it available to everyone." His mission is to bring the papaya enzyme "into" everyone on a daily basis: "I have become accustomed to a level of joy and health that I don't want to lose!"

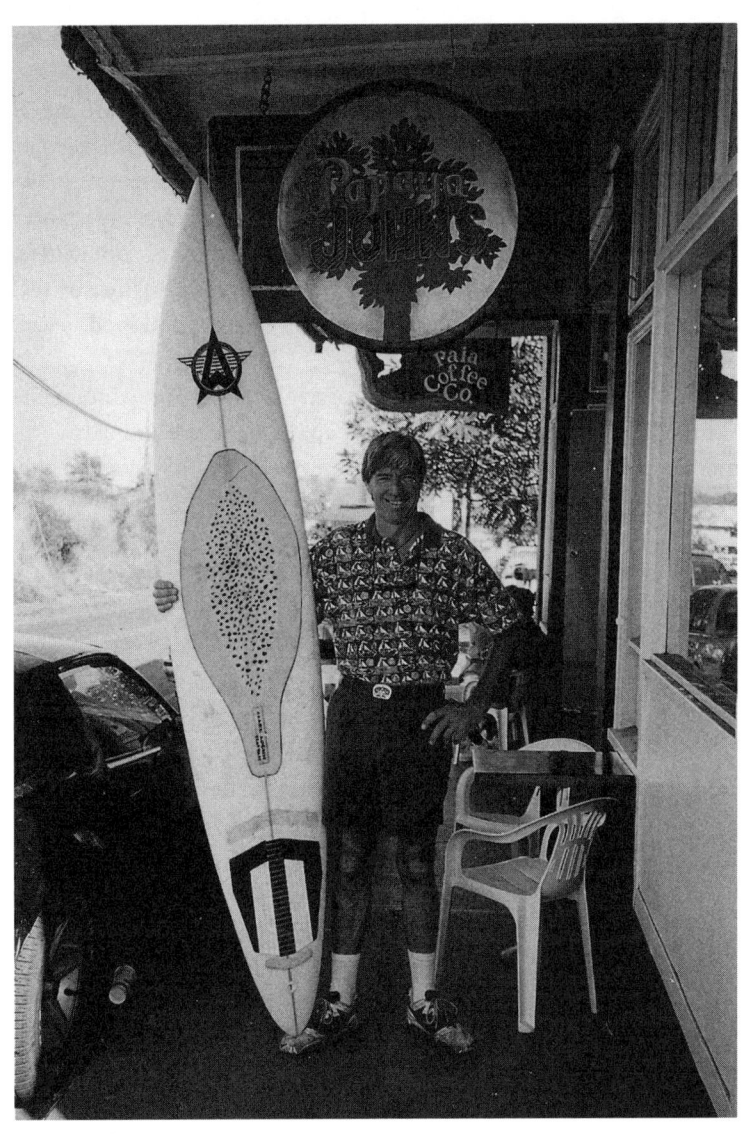

Papaya John

The source material for his products are guaranteed organically grown papayas that are harvested during the period of greatest enzyme activity. His range of products includes various papaya bars, granulates from green papaya, and a dressing from papaya seeds.

John raises the papayas himself, which sometimes contain double the normal amount of enzyme and are resistant to virus diseases.

John plans to start an organic papaya farm in Peru in order to make it possible for the farmers there to buy their land back. Perhaps he will move to Costa Rica himself in order to obtain less expensive raw materials for his papaya products. In his garden on Maui, papayas grow to a size of 22 pounds. He wouldn't think of living somewhere where papayas don't grow. Every day, John drinks papaya juice by the quart: "A fantastic possibility to feel fit and be in a good mood even when fasting!"

On Maui, this juice can be purchased frozen in pint containers. When John travels, he takes enough papaya granulate and bars with him to continually fill his enzyme reserves. "I'm addicted to the papaya enzyme," John says with his infectious laugh.

A Papaya Meditation

If you purchased this book or had it given to you, you are probably already in contact with the deva, the spirit of the papaya plant. There are no coincidences. If you consciously want to develop a closer contact with the papaya deva, you should spend as much time as possible with the plant. For example, I give my Colombian mountain papayas in the garden first and second degree Authentic Reiki in order to support them in this climate that is foreign to them. In addition, I often treat them with the universal energy and talk to them.

Plants are very receptive to vibrations, which includes the vibrations of love in particular. If you seek a deep contact with exotic plants, you should travel to their home in the tropics and meditate there with them for a longer period of time. In their native surroundings, the plants are stronger and more "self-confident." You can sit under a papaya tree or lean against the trunk; then place one hand over your solar plexus and the other hand on the opposite side of the back with its palm against the tree. You can also take the fruit in your hands, close your eyes, and meditate about the gifts that it has waiting for you.

When you meditate with the papaya, become empty in order to perceive and absorb the vibrations and mood of the tree. Pay attention to the inspirations it may give you. In order to strengthen your resonance with the papaya tree, eat a great deal of papayas. You can nourish yourself exclusively from the papaya for a few days!

When you eat, close your eyes and focus your meditative consciousness on the plant: its taste and its effect on your body and soul. You don't need to wait until the fruit is digested because the subtle information is already absorbed and evaluated in the mouth. For example, right after eating you may feel lighter, more vivacious, and clearer! I have discovered that papaya not only brightens my mood but also clarifies my thoughts. Apparently, it is meant to be "food for the soul" and contains not only bioactive but also psychoactive substances. The latter have not yet been discovered, but they still work anyway.

Fruit should be eaten only on an empty stomach and without other foods—as a mono diet—when meditating. People who eat raw plant foods or nourish themselves primarily from these raw foods probably have the deepest experiences of eating enjoyment. For example, the durian fruit from Thailand is "heaven on earth" for the raw-food eater, while it is often perceived to be a "stinky fruit" by those who eat mixed foods.

If you have perceptions while meditating with the plant or eating its fruit, trust them, no matter how subtle they may be. Your own authentic experiences are much more valuable than any second-hand knowledge, regardless of how good the books may be. Even if you do not perceive very much at the beginning, the information from the plant has an effect on your subconscious mind. So don't be discouraged! Perhaps the papaya will send you "messages" in dreams or some other form of knowledge later.

Once you have discovered your love of this plant, you might develop the desire to collect stories, fairytales, and legends that involved the papaya. These legends are not just fantasies but form vivid depictions of what native peoples have perceived as the reality of the plant's spirit. You can also meditate on them, comprehending and interpreting the groups of images.

Or you can collect pictures and recipes for the papaya and develop your own ways of preparing it. There are no limits set for your imagination. Perhaps you might also want to make your own ointments and masks from a papaya basis, flower essences, or fragrant oils (also see the recipes you can make in *The Papaya in Beauty Care* on page 149).

In addition to the many impulses I have received from the people of the Findhorn Foundation for developing a deep connection to plants, I have also been inspired by ethno-physician Dr. Wolf-Dieter Storl. This author writes beautiful German-language books about plant divas (the goddess and her plant angels: the art of healing, cultural history, mythology and folk religion) and holds seminars teaching a meditative approach to plants.

Among other things, the Aborigines use the flowers of the papaya to come in contact with their higher selves before making important decisions. The blossoms smell seductively sweet, similar to lilies of the valley, and lead us to spheres of higher consciousness. You can make a cold infusion from the blossoms and use them, like Bach flowers, to expand your consciousness. Or make massage oils, aroma oils (for aroma lamps), or your own perfumes.

Incense sticks with the fragrance of papaya are available from Maroma, and possibly other companies. I hope that the robust Colombian mountain papaya from the Andes will soon spread in the cooler climates: Health-conscious people and plant-lovers are invited to plant it in their gardens, balconies, and flower containers (see *Growing Your Own Papayas* on page 42 ff).

Books and Articles about Papayas

The selection of papaya books has been quite limited in the past. There have only been four books in English up to now, of which two are out of print:

A rich source of information for papaya fans is the book by Chester D. French: *Papaya—the Melon of Health*. The author does not hide his enthusiasm for papayas and has been involved with them for much of his life. Many trips took him to papaya countries like Mexico and Tanzania. Sometimes a bit wordy, French explains the health benefits and medical significance of the papaya to his readers. He also has many tips for those who want to cultivate papayas themselves. His chapter about the papaya enzyme papain and the description of the many possibilities for applying it for health and beauty purposes are still relevant. When I read the book, I wondered why all the advantages of the papaya, which have been used in the USA since the beginning of the 20th century, are neglected in Europe. I hope that French's book will soon be available again.

An oddity, which is not available either, is the book by Dr. Thomas Lucas: *To the Medical Profession, Scientists and Thinkers: the Most Wonderful Tree in the World, the Papaw Tree (Carica Papaya)*. Dr. Lucas was a physician and botanist. At the beginning of the 20th century, he recognized the healing power of the papaya and believed that he has found the greatest healing remedy in the world. In Brisbane, Australia, he directed a hospital called "Vera," in which patients were treated exclusively with the papaya remedies that he developed.

Dr. Lucas was exuberant about the success in healing severe cases that had been given up by orthodox medicine, such as cancer. Even if everything that he said is not one-hundred percent correct, the examples are still very impressive. The effects of the papaya preparations that Dr. Lucas had developed were also verified by London's Great Ormond Street Hospital (published in the London *Medical Magazine* in May 1910). According to this research, many operations were spared through the use of papaya. His "Lucas Papaw Ointment" remedy is still sold under the name of "Vera Papaw Hospital" by his grandchildren in Australia, who are attempting to export this product to Europe and the USA.

A useful guide for papaya-growers is the little book by Paul O'Hare: *Growing Papaws in South Queensland*. Here we learn everything about the required investment of capital for a papaya farm, selecting the right kind of papayas, developing the plantation, choosing the seeds, fertilizer, watering, controlling weeds, using mulches, possible diseases and how to fight them, harvesting papayas, packing and selling them. A calendar provides a summary of which work needs to be done and when. Unfortunately, the topic of organic papaya cultivation is treated somewhat briefly. All in all, it is a useful guide for anyone who lives in a subtropical climate and wants to establish an existence based on papayas.

As previously mentioned, there is also a book on the papaya by Harald Tietze: *Papaya (Pawpaw), The Medicine Tree*. It contains much detailed information about the use of papayas by the Aborigines (also see *Papaya as Australia's Cancer-Healing "Remedy."* on page 109).

In view of the limited literature selection, I would like to comment on a few articles about papayas: An article on the cultivation and use of papaya by Gerhard Küthe and Hajo Spoehase in the German-language magazine *Der Tropenlandwirt* (The Tropical Farmer) provides information about the versatile possibilities for using the **papaya as a "cash crop" for developing nations**. This would help them pay for fertilizer and farm feed so that the poorest inhabitants of rural areas can be helped.

A somewhat older article on "Papaya" by John J. Miller in the *Northwest Technocrat* praises its properties as a digestive aid and antacid remedy.

Recipes for the Kitchen

Many people eat papaya with Parmesan ham, in chicken salad, with cottage cheese, or in drinks with gin and peppermint liqueur. Since I am a vegetarian and don't drink alcohol, I have largely omitted recipes with milk products, alcohol, and meat for nutritional-physiological reasons (see *Help against Acidosis* on page 77). However, here is one tip: Papaya in, with, or after protein dishes including meat or cheese makes them easier to digest!

These recipes should be understood as suggestions and there are no limits set for your imagination. Papaya tastes good and fits with almost all kinds of dishes, so give them a try! Papayas alone are delicious, and you can also drip lemon juice onto them.

The seeds can be dried, ground, and used like pepper. Like the ripe fruit, they not only contain a great deal of vitamin C but also the enzyme papain, which quickly digests protein, fat, and starch.

In tropical countries, the papaya is already eaten at breakfast along with other fruits, such as the pineapple, to stimulate digestion. The young leaves or papaya sprouts can be added to salad, making it even more nutritious since papaya leaves contain more papain, beta carotene, and vitamin C than the ripe fruit. In addition, never throw away the skin: cut it into small pieces and add them to salad or use them to make papaya vinegar for dressings. They can also be used for cosmetic purposes (see recipes in *The Papaya in Beauty Care* on page 149 ff).

In the South Seas, the unripe fruit is cooked together with finely chopped peanuts and served as a side dish. Many Moslems break their daily fast during Rammadan with "mamboga": Unripe papayas are cooked and made into a paste with finely chopped peanuts, salt, and chilies.

When there is a surplus on the market, ripe papayas can sometimes be purchased on sale: peel them, cut them into pieces, and dry them in the oven at the lowest temperature. Stick a wooden spoon in the oven door to allow the air to circulate. A fruit dryer (dehydrator) is also useful for this purpose. You can adjust the temperature very precisely and even dry papaya seeds. Dried papayas taste very good; they even have a more intense taste than the fresh fruit. Children and adults appreciate them as a snack while traveling, hiking, or at school or college.

Dried fruit can also be purchased in health food stores and natural food stores. Be sure that the fruit has not been treated with sulfur or sugar. Also ask if it was dried in tropical lands at temperatures below 122 degrees Fahrenheit and not in the sun. Otherwise, its vitamins and enzymes may be lost. In order to activate the enzymes, you can soak the dried papaya in water over night.

When I travel and don't know if I can get papaya at my destination, I take along the green papaya granulate (from organic cultivation, which can be obtained from Papaya John) and flour made of ground papaya seeds as an alternative to fresh fruit. The granulate must be softened for twenty minutes before using it. Very tasty!

PAPAYA DREAM
Use eight dried apricot halves (not treated with sulfur), one large apple, one half of a papaya that has been peeled and cut into pieces. Soak the apricots over night (and save the water to drink later). Juice from the apple and papaya. Add the juice to the apricots and mix everything in a mixer or juicer at a medium speed. Enjoy either alone or as a dressing for fruit salad.

PINA COLADA
Use two cups of fresh pineapple, one half of a papaya that has been peeled and cut into pieces, two cups of freshly grated coconut, and one cup of water (as desired). Juice the pineapple and the papaya. Mix all ingredients for two minutes at the highest speed. Then strain and serve with a slice of lemon and a mint leaf.

PAPAYA SALSA
Mix three cups of grated papaya, a cup of grated sweet red hot peppers, one teaspoon of lemon juice, one teaspoon of honey, and a pinch of ground red pepper. Eat with tortillas or rice—or as a dip for raw vegetables.

PAPAYA PUDDING
Stir papaya fruit granulate with the recommended amount of water or red beet juice and mix with one to two teaspoons of psyllium husks (available at natural food stores). Let mixture sit for 20 minutes. If desired, the pudding can be sweetened with honey.

PAPAYA ASPIC
Peel one ripe papaya and remove the seeds. (You can plant them, use them for cleansing the intestine, and as a digestive aid. Or chew them dried against worms, grind them like pepper and mix with water, or use as pepper in salad, etc.) Cut the ripe papaya into

pieces and liquefy in a mixer or juicer. Add one lemon for two cups of papaya. You can also add a bit of honey, if you like. Fill the mixture into a glass container and put in the refrigerator. After a few hours, the papaya will solidify into "papaya aspic." Eat it alone or with meals.

PAPAYA PUDDING II
Mix the papayas from the glass container with juice, one teaspoon of psyllium husks, one teaspoon of either acerola cherry powder, ascorbic acid, or lemon juice and allow to stand for 20 minutes. Can also be topped with whipped cream.
You can also use fresh papayas for this recipe by liquefying half of the fruit in a mixer. As an alternative: Let dried papayas soak overnight and use as above.

ASIATIC PAPAYA SALAD
For this vegetarian salad, you need two green or half-green papayas, two medium-sized tomatoes, one-half cup of peanuts, approx. two tablespoons of maple syrup, three cloves of garlic, four tablespoons of lime juice, three tablespoons of light soy sauce, and, if you like it spicy, three chilies.
Use a cucumber grater to grate the papayas into fine strips. Cube the tomatoes. Crush the garlic with a fork, cut the chilies into small pieces, and mix with the other ingredients. Add the papayas and tomatoes to the mixture and serve.

"SOUTH-SEA MAGIC" SALAD
For six portions, you will need one large pineapple, one soft mango, one firm papaya, two ripe star fruit (carambola), three bananas, 250 grams of lychees (fresh, if possible!), and the juice of one lemon. Cut the fruit into small pieces and drip the lemon juice onto it. This salad is a vitamin and enzyme "bomb"!

PAPAYA FRUIT SHERBET
If you find papayas on sale that are very ripe: peel and cut them into pieces, then freeze in airtight containers.

With a (Champion) juicer, you can make wonderful fruit sherbets from the frozen fruit. Puree equal portions of papaya and pineapple and freeze. An alternative: puree ripe papayas in a mixer, add lemon or lime juice according to taste, and freeze.

PAPAYA APPLESAUCE

Papaya applesauce is a nice change for breakfast and children like it as well. Take one-half cup of freshly squeezed apple juice or one-half cup of water. Peel two large apples and cut into quarters. Mix together with one-half teaspoon of cinnamon or nutmeg (or a quarter teaspoon of each). Add one fresh or frozen banana and one-half of a papaya (or two very ripe, soft date plums). Puree in a mixer until the sauce is smooth. Recipe makes one to two portions.

PAPAYA FRUIT DIP

Puree in a mixer: one-half of a papaya, one-quarter cup of fresh orange juice, and a pinch of nutmeg or vanilla. Serve this fruit dip with fruit or on top of it.

FILLED PAPAYA

For this recipe, you will need one onion, two tablespoons of sunflower oil, one half pound of natural rice, a vegetable-soup broth cube, one package (one pound) of frozen giant deep-sea shrimp, lemon juice, two papayas, one package of light sauce (hollandaise), two tablespoons of sweet cream, and two ounces of grated Gouda.

Peel the onion and cut in cubes. Heat the oil and fry the onion cubes in it until glassy. Add rice and braise briefly. Add four cups of water and vegetable-soup cube. Bring to a boil and let cook gently in a closed pan for about 40 minutes at low heat. Thaw the shrimps, sprinkle with lemon juice, and mix with the rice. Wash the papaya, peel, cut in half, and remove the seeds with a spoon. Fill with the shrimp rice. Place the remaining rice in a baking dish and put the filled papayas on top of it.

Heat one cup of water. Stir in the light sauce and boil for one minute. Stir in the sweet cream and Gouda cheese. Pour this sauce over the papayas and bake in the oven at 400 degrees Fahrenheit for about 15 minutes.

PAPAYA CHILI SAUCE

For this spicy sauce, you will need two tablespoons of finely cut chili, one-quarter of a papaya chopped into small pieces, 2 ounces of raisins, one half of a finely chopped onion, three pressed garlic cloves, one-half teaspoon of ground turmeric, and 2 fluid ounces of vinegar.

You can either prepare this sauce raw in a mixer or cook while stirring constantly and then puree. Put the remaining sauce into a tightly closed glass container (papain attacks plastic) in the refrigerator. This sauce is delicious as a dip for corn chips or potato chips or with fresh carrot sticks.

MILLI BRASILLI

This exotic milk cocktail is served in the restaurant of the Alpamare Hotel on Lake Zurich. It consists of a mixture of papaya/guanabana with a mild yogurt made from skim milk, sweet whey, cream, butter milk—and the vitamins E, B6, B2, and B12—with only 4.5 percent fat in the milk portion and without preservatives. When making this yourself, I suggest omitting the vitamins since there are plenty of them in the papaya!

PAPAYA CREAM

Cut a well-ripened papaya in half, remove the seeds, and remove the fruit pulp with a spoon. Puree together with the juice of a fresh grapefruit in a mixer or juicer. Carefully stir in stiff whipped cream and serve in a dessert glass with a spoon of cream on the top.

An alternative: Instead of stiff whipped cream, you can puree it with vanilla ice cream (also available made from soy beans and honey).

PAPAYA DRINK I

You will need two ripe papayas, two teaspoons of lemon juice, two teaspoons of honey, and some powdered ginger. Cut the papaya into cubes and divide among four glasses. Top it with a pinch of powdered ginger, sprinkle the cubes with lemon juice and honey, and fill up the glasses with mineral water or soda water. Serve with straws.

PAPAYA DRINK II
Mix equal quantities of pineapple and papaya juice.

PAPAYA FRUIT CUP
You will need one ripe papaya, one piece of watermelon (about 1/8), and one small honeydew melon, as well as Benedictine or Grand Marnier, 1-2 tablespoons of raw sugar or maple syrup, 1/2 cup of whipped cream, and vanilla sugar.
Use a melon scooper to carve out round balls of papaya and melon. Fill four Champagne glasses with the orange, green, and red balls; sprinkle with liqueur and some maple syrup or raw sugar. Top each glass with whipped cream and vanilla sugar.

PAPAYA FRUIT SALAD I
Peel and cut the ripe papaya into cubes. Add pineapple cubes, slices of banana, and fresh or thawed (frozen) raspberries, gooseberries, or red currants. Season with lemon juice and pour papaya puree or some maple syrup over the fruit.

PAPAYA FRUIT SALAD II
Mix pieces of ripe papaya with banana slices and mango cubes. Add lemon or lime juice according to taste.

PAPAYA SAUERKRAUT
In the Philippines, people pickle green, shredded papaya with onions and pepper pods in vinegar.

PAPAYA SAUCE
Peel the unripe fruit, remove the seeds, and cut the fruit into cubes. Then cook in a little water with sugar (alternatives: maple syrup or honey) with (organic) lemon or lime peel, ginger, cloves, and cinnamon until soft.

PAPAYA MARMELADE
For two pounds of green papayas that already have yellow fruit pulp, you will need 1-1/2 pounds of raw sugar and one lemon cut in small pieces. Cut the papayas into cubes and cook together with the other ingredients until the desired consistency is reached.
You can also make marmalade using mangos or pineapple in a 1:1 ratio with the papaya.

The Papaya as a Healing Remedy

The green, somewhat unripe papaya and the leaves and the seeds of the ripe papaya used for therapeutic purposes. Examples of these are: dissolving tumors and cancer cells (see section on this topic), against arteriosclerosis, rheumatism, osteoporosis, intervertebral disk problems due to chondrosis (see *Papaya for Backaches—Chemonucleolysis and More* on page 126), acidosis (see *Help against Acidosis* on page 77), diabetics, chronic digestive problems, bronchitis, asthma, inflammations, skin problems, cellulite, overweight, high blood pressure, and cardiac insufficiency.

If you eat food that is lacking in enzymes, you should get used to chewing peeled papaya slices with it or spicing it with powder from the papaya seeds. The enzymes stimulate the activity of the pancreas and accelerate the decomposition of difficult-to-digest proteins found in meat, fish, cheese, pizzas, eggs, etc. Digestion is stimulated and the acid-alkali equilibrium balanced.

As an alternative, you can dry fruit that is still fairly firm (see *Recipes for the Kitchen* on page 160) to make an ideal nutritional supplement when away from home. Dried, unripe papayas taste better than the fresh fruit and need no seasoning to improve their taste.

ANTI-ACID DRINK
Add the juice of one-half pound of papaya to one pint of water and one pint of fresh celery or cucumber juice. This drink also aids in eliminating waste deposits and excess weight.

PAPAYA TEA

This very valuable digestant tea, which contains a large amount of vitamin C, can be prepared from the seeds of green and ripe papayas. Gently boil one-quarter cup of seeds with two quarts of water for about half an hour. Then filter and season with ginger or cayenne pepper. If you wish, you can add lemon juice. This tea is recommended for dissolving deposits. Ideally, drinks a large quantity (one quart) one hour after eating papaya in the form of sauce or herbs.
I find that papaya tea and "Classic Yogi Tea" taste good together. Simply boil the seeds with the given amount of water and two flat tablespoons of Yogi Tea, then filter. You can also prepare a tea from papaya leaves. In addition to stimulating digestion, this tea supposedly prevents and heals cancer.

PAPAYA VEGETABLES

As a side dish, the green papaya makes meat more tender and easier to digest. Cut it into pieces without the seeds and cook with meat or poultry. Papaya vegetables are also recommended as a side dish for fish or hard-to-digest proteins and fats.
In the West Indies, young papaya leaves are cooked and eaten like spinach.

PAPAYA "PEPPER"

The dark seeds of the ripe fruit, like the fruit pulp of the green papaya, are reported to contain inhibiting substances against cancer and fungus. Moreover, they are a good medication for eliminating and preventing worms. Chew about 20 to 30 of the ripe seeds well; the remaining seed should be dried by simply placing a plate of them on the heater. The dried seeds can be finely ground in a coffee or pepper mill and used as seasoning for soups, salads, and dips.

PAPAYA JUICE

The juice of the ripe papaya stimulates digestion and glandular functioning (see *Papaya as a Digestive Aid* on page 91). It tastes delicious alone or mixed with fresh pineapple juice. The indestructible "Champion Juicer" has proved to have the highest yield.

The juice of the green papaya also has great therapeutic value, especially against chronic inflammation, waste deposits in the intestine, weak glands, tumors, hyperacidity, excess fat, and cellulite. Use the entire fruit without seeds, but with the skin (one-half to one pound per person) and juice it. Then mix the juice with one pint of freshly squeezed apple or vegetable juice. Its taste is too bitter alone and the effect is too intensive. One recommendation is to drink one pint of non-carbonated water, green tea, or herb tea one-half hour before taking the papaya juice or herbs in the morning.

When you use a juicer, you can store the fiber pulp, keeping it moist and cool, and use as a tasty raw food (see below *Papaya Herb*). Like all freshly squeezed juices, papaya juice should always be consumed immediately to avoid loss of vitamins and enzymes. Do not use any plastic containers to store green papaya juice because papain attacks plastic.

If you don't have a juicer, you can grate the green papaya without seeds like an apple, mix with freshly grated apple or ripe papaya, and chew thoroughly.

Depending on the amount of waste substances in the body, excess weight, or cellulite, you can consume one-half pound of green papaya as juice (diluted 1:1) or pureed as a meal three times a day.

PAPAYA–APPLE HERB

Cut a medium-sized (about one pound) green to yellow-green papaya in half. Store one of the halves well covered on a porcelain or glass plate in the refrigerator. Peel off the bitter skin of the other half. Only include the skin in diets against cancer or intense waste deposits in the body. Then cube the peeled papaya and two peeled Boskop apples (Boskop has the highest vitamin C content of the various apple types). Liquefy the apples with half a cup of water or apple juice (1/8 l) in an electric mixer. Then add the papaya pieces without seeds (dry for pepper or tea!) to the electric mixer and make into sauce.

To remove waste substances from the lymph and respiratory system, you can add 1-2 teaspoons of freshly peeled horseradish or fresh ginger can be added.

The mixture can also be seasoned with finely ground fennel seeds, anise, or licorice.

PAPAYA HERB I, TART AND SPICY
Prepare the green to yellow-green papayas, which are still hard and contain the valuable enzyme papain, in a manner similar to the papaya-apple herb. Liquefy the cubed pieces together with one-half cup of sauerkraut, red beet, or pineapple juice. Then mix in two tablespoons of cold-pressed olive oil (first pressing) with freshly squeezed horseradish and a pinch of salt. If you use red beet juice, mildly acidify the herb with one or two teaspoons of liquid whey. Then pour the olive-oil mixture over the papaya herb.

As an alternative to vegetable or fruit juice, you can remove the juice from a ripe lemon, dilute with one-half cup of water, and then combine with the olive oil, salt, and spices. You can keep the three daily portions of this in an airtight glass or porcelain container in the refrigerator, but not for more than one day.

Halima Neumann believes she healed herself from cancer with papaya juice and papaya herb (see *Case example: Halima Neumann's Papaya Therapy* on page 106).

PAPAYA HERB II
Remove the seeds from a hard papaya, grate the papaya with its skin or liquefy it in a mixer. An alternative: papaya fruit granulate. Add freshly squeezed orange or lemon juice and season with lemon, garlic, or ground dark papaya seeds.

PAPAYA FRUIT GRANULATE
To remove waste substances from the intestine and deacidify the body, take two to three tablespoons of papaya fruit granulate (Papaya John), which is made by carefully drying organically grown green papaya at 122 degrees Fahrenheit. Dissolve the granulate in one cup of warm water, fruit juice, or vegetable juice and allow it to absorb water for one-half hour.

I get the best taste with apple, red beet, or carrot juice. Add papaya-seed powder to intensify the waste-removal effect.

If you want to pep up the pleasant-tasting granulate, you can add grated apples, pineapples, or grapefruit (grown organically, if you want to support the healing effects). If your stomach is overly acidic, don't add any fruit juice. One exception: the non-acidic ripe papaya fruit.

For **detoxification of the liver:** Combine the papaya fruit granulate or homemade papaya herb with a mixture of dandelion and red beet, sauerkraut, or artichoke juice. After the granulate has absorbed the water, add finely grated horseradish.

An alternative: Use celery (or red beet) juice for soaking and then one to two tablespoons of barley-grass powder and one teaspoon of papaya-seed powder. Let it soak for five more minutes, then chew well!

For **diarrhea:** Soak papaya fruit granulate or homemade papaya herb in an equal portion of diluted concentrated blueberry juice (health food store), then stir in two tablespoons of active calcium (pharmacy) and let soak for another ten minutes.

For **fungal infestation:** Let the granulate soak in warm vegetable broth or mix the homemade papaya herb with vegetable broth. You can also use vegetable juice, diluted concentrated fruit juice (from blackberries, for example) without sugar, or diluted applesauce. Season with papaya-seed powder, ginger, garlic or horseradish.

To **remove waste substances from veins, blood, and lymph:** Add freshly grated horseradish and a slightly sour apple, such as Boskop, to presoaked granulate or homemade papaya herb.

As a **vermicide (remedy against worms)**, A. Vogel recommends a preventive worm treatment once a year, which can also be used in acute cases: Every day for three weeks, chew one tablespoon of papaya seeds from the ripe fruit or dry and ground seeds to spread over dishes as powder.

In cases of parasite infestation, this treatment should be repeated after a three-week pause since papain kills the worms but not the eggs. Repeat this treatment until there is no more evidence of worms. Another alternative is to eat papaya herb made of unripe papaya, possibly mixed with grated carrots and seasoned with lemon juice. Raw carrots expel intestinal parasites (also see extra chapter on this topic).

As a **cancer remedy:** Halima Neumann writes in her book on stopping cancer that she recovered from the disease after unsuccessful chemotherapy by drinking green-papaya juice and eating papaya herb (see corresponding chapters for details).

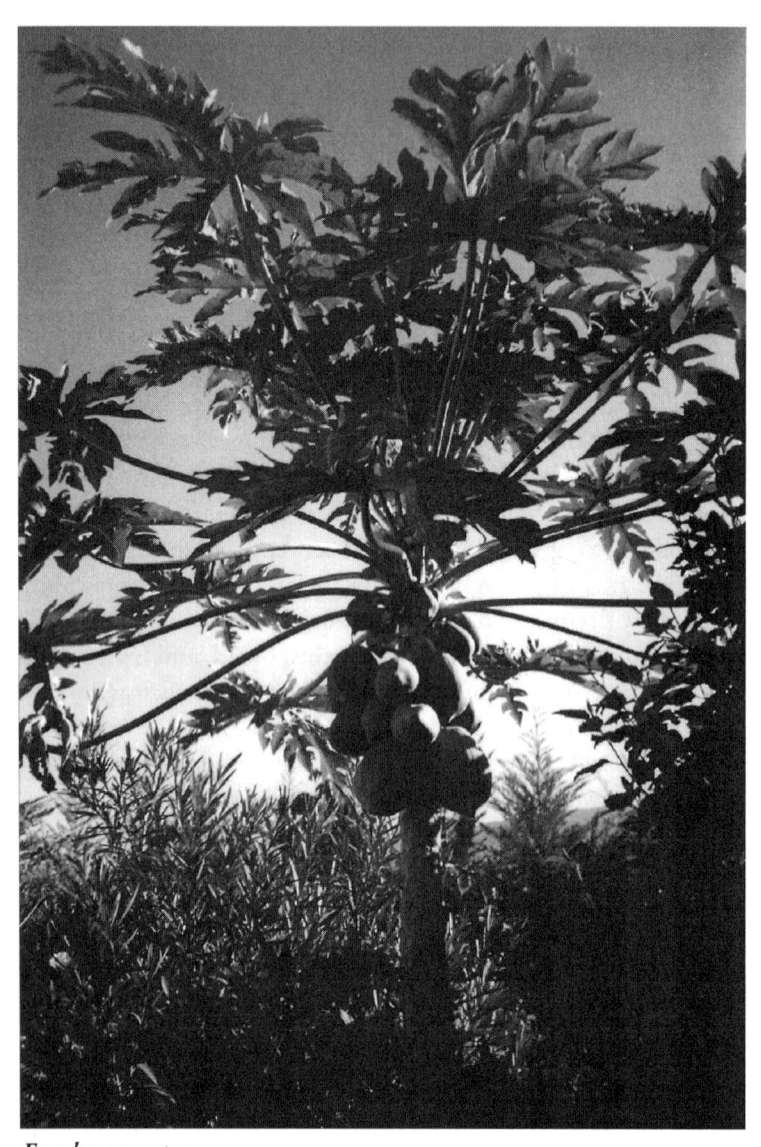

Female papaya tree

Papaya—Healing from A to Z

Experience has shown that papaya is effective (and also useful as preventive treatment) in the following situations. For serious health disorders, you should naturally always consult a specialist!

ACIDOSIS

There is hardly a human being today who does not suffer from hyperacidity. Chronic diseases require an "acidic basis"! Together with a basic change in our nutrition and life style, the papaya—as a fruit that is extremely alkali forming when metabolized—can help us to once again achieve an acid-alkali equilibrium. Examples of "acidic diseases" are rheumatism, diabetes, arthrosis, and cancer. Additional information on this topic can be found in *Help against Acidosis* on page 77 ff.

ADRENAL GLANDS

The adrenal glands are not only decisively involved in states of agitation and our emotions in general: They also stimulate the muscles and the nervous system, taking care of repairs and the renewal of cell and tissue structures. In addition, the adrenal glands are "a true cornucopia of hormones": They create almost four dozen different hormone types. Consequently, our glandular system and the adrenal glands don't need just need any kind of nutrients but nutritious food like fresh, raw fruit juices and vegetable juices. Eating ripe papayas contributes greatly to maintaining balance in the activity of the adrenal glands.

AGING, PREMATURE

Papaya can slow down the aging process and rejuvenate us (see *REJUVENATION* and *Papaya—A Fountain of Youth* on page 69).

AIDS

Under the title of "New Hope for AIDS," Anthony J. Cichoke *(Enzymes and Enzyme Therapy)* describes successes in enzyme therapy for AIDS patients in the USA Australia, and Costa Rica. In most cases, death is caused by the destruction of the helper cells by the immune complexes, which leads to a breakdown of the defense system. This is where enzyme therapy takes action: the protein-splitting enzymes are able to bring the immune complexes back into the blood circulation and dissolve them. The result: The patient remains HIV-positive but becomes free of the symptoms. Enzyme therapy arrests the disease in the early stage, activates helper cells, and prevents infectious diseases and malignant tumors.

ALCOHOL

In tropical countries and on the islands of the South Sea, papayas are eaten after drinking alcohol in order to reduce the negative effects—hangover and headaches. However, this tip isn't meant to increase your consumption of alcohol! If you wish to live a healthy lifestyle in the long run, only use alcohol very sparingly or, even better drop the alcohol habit in order to prevent hyperacidity and other health problems. The substances in red wine that prevent heart attacks and possibly cancer are also found in red and orange-colored fruits such as red grapes and papaya.

Mexican beer is now sold as "health beer" because papain, the most important papaya enzyme, is used in its production. This is deceptive advertising since the fresh fruit has much higher concentrations than any industrially produced products.

ALLERGIES

The theme of "allergies" is very complex and the problem is gaining in explosiveness. One-fifth of all children suffer from food allergies and other allergies! One of the main causes is false nutrition and the related "protein waste" in the intestine. Papayas and enzyme remedies containing papain could be a great help here (see *Allergies—When the "Barrel" is Full!* on page 111 ff).

AMEBIC DYSENTERY

Grind the seeds of a ripe papaya and take one teaspoon of them in warm water every three hours at the first sign of symptoms. As an alternative: Chew the seeds, take "Papayasan" or another product containing papain. This treatment is only effective as long as the amebas are not yet in the liver.

Vogel recommends eating papaya seeds or leaves, or two tablets of Papayasan or other Papaya Enzymes, after meals in tropical lands as a preventive treatment. French advises taking two teaspoons of papaya seeds in honey or syrup every six hours.

ANIMALS

In veterinary medicine, enzymes have become indispensable for fighting viruses. Dr. R. Dunkel added enzymes to the dry food of chickens suffering from a vicious leucosis in Chad (Africa). In contrast to untreated animals, all of which died, almost every chicken treated with enzymes recovered. The German handbook of pharmaceutical practice written by Hager recommends a cold papaya infusion as a digestant for horses.

In countries such as India and Jamaica, papaya is used as animal feed. In the German city of Landshut, the veterinarian Dr. Heinz Glock helped enzyme therapy to make a breakthrough. He proved that enzymes had amazing results in fighting the dangerous horse and pig croup and even cattle pneumonia, which is often deadly. In one case, he cured 240 cows within two to five days.

Currently, tests on the effect of papain on udder infections in cows are being carried out at the University of Leipzig.

APPETITE

A tea ("Pap Tea") from papaya leaves, which stimulates the appetite, is available in the USA and Australia. You can also make a tea from the seeds (see *Recipes for the Kitchen* on page 160). The ripe papaya or its freshly squeezed juice has a similar effect. (Further recipes are in *The Papaya in the Folk Medicine of India* on page 137 ff).

ARTERIOSCLEROSIS

See *HEART.*

ARTHRITIS, ARTHROSIS

Papain has been successfully used together with other enzymes as a preventive treatment and therapy for joint inflammation and the appearance of attrition, as well as internally and externally in the form of ointments (also see *Papaya against Inflammation* on page 115).

ASTHMA
The Indians in Mexico cook fresh (or dried) papaya leaves with a pint of water and strain the liquid. Then they drink the hot broth mornings and evenings in small sips (also see *Papaya in Native Central and South American Plant Therapy* on page 133).

BACKACHES
According to Dr. Hoffmann, an alkaline-based nutrition can help stop the deterioration of the vertebrae. Papaya helps us regain our acid-alkali equilibrium.

Halima Neuman assumes that cartilage can be regenerated through papain (see *REJUVENATION* and *Papaya for Backaches—Chemonucleolysis and More* on page 126). Physical exercise also improves the circulation and nutrition of the cartilage and joints. Leibold recommends internal and external use of combination enzyme preparations for backaches, joint inflammation, and the appearance of attrition.

BAD BREATH
Bad breath is very often the result of digestive disorder. Papaya enzyme tablets are recommended as an excellent remedy for better digestion. In addition, you can take Lactaid tablets against milk allergy.

BIRTH CONTROL
See *CONTRACEPTIVES*.

BLOOD PRESSURE
"Pap tea", a tea from papaya leaves, has a mild blood-pressure regulating effect as a result of its low carpaine content. Eating the ripe fruit pulp of the papaya has proved useful in lowering high blood pressure by diluting the blood and relieving the heart. (Also see *The Papaya in Native Central and South American Plant Therapy* on page 133, as well as *The Folk Medicine of India* on page 137). This blood-pressure lowering effect has also been observed when enzyme preparations containing papain are taken (also see *HEART*).

BRONCHITIS
For bronchitis, the Central American Indians drink a decoction from the papaya leaves: Boil the papaya leaves in one pint of water

and then strain. Drink this decoction in small portions hot and in sips, twice a day: after getting up and before going to bed (see *The Papaya in Native Central and South American Plant Therapy* on page 133, as well as *The Papaya in the Folk Medicine of India* on page 137). Enzyme preparations also help to end a bronchial infection more quickly.

BRUISES
See *SPRAINS*.

BURNS
Apply papain to remove dead tissue. If the wound burns after applying an enzyme ointment, dilute it with water. You can also use the milk juice of the unripe fruit. If applied immediately after a burn, no blisters will form (see *The Papaya in Native Central and South American Plant Therapy* on page 133, as well as *The Papaya in the Folk Medicine of India* on page 137).

CANCER
For centuries, the South American Indians have used the leaves and fruits of the papaya plant for cancer sores, thereby becoming the instinctive founders of enzyme therapy against cancer. The kahunas of Hawaii and the Aborigines in Australia use the papaya as a healing plant (see corresponding *The Papaya in the Ethno-Medicine of Native Peoples* on page 132).

Today, enzyme preparations are successfully used as preventive treatment and therapy for cancer patients. For cancer prevention, enzymes combined with a sensible, healthy lifestyle are unbeatable. Further information can be found in *Cancer—Causes and Alternatives* on page 95 and *Papain in Enzyme Therapy against Cancer* on page 103.

CANDIDA
See *FUNGI*.

CELIAC DISEASE
See *GLUTEN INTOLERANCE*.

CELLULITE

When cellulite appears, the connective tissue has been changed as a result of metabolic disturbances. Consequently, creams and lotions don't help! Recommendations for a successful battle against cottage-cheese skin are physical exercise and an enzyme-rich diet with metabolically active fruits such as papaya, kiwi, and pineapple.

CHRONIC FATIGUE SYNDROME (CFS)

The chronic fatigue syndrome is probably triggered by the Type-6 Herpes virus and is found in more than two million patients in the US alone, most of whom are between 25 and 40 years of age. It is thought that the extreme tiredness results when the virus gets into the central nervous system. Enzyme therapy is capable of activating the natural killer cells of the immune system. In addition to enzymes, vitamins (A, E, and D) and thymus-gland preparations have been used successfully. This success indicates that false nutrition plays a role in causing the illness: CFS patients are certain to have had a diet that wasn't rich enough in enzyme and vitamins, which results in a weakening of the immune system.

COLITIS

In internal medicine, medication containing papain with bismuth is used against intestinal infections such as diarrhea, irritable colon, and colitis (chronic large intestinal infection). In India, the seeds are administered against inflammation of the mucosa of the digestive tract because they contain antibacterial substances

COLDS, FLU

Papayas have already been used for centuries, both internally and externally, against colds and flu. They strengthen our immune system as a preventive treatment (see *Papaya—Help for Colds and Flu* on page 113). Papaya enzyme tablets reduce the swelling in sinusitis and bronchitis and clear out bacteria and mucous in the affected area. Recommended dosage: Let the tablets slowly dissolve in your mouth four times a day.

CONSTIPATION

Large quantities of papaya fruit act against constipation as a mild laxative without side effects. If you also want to activate your digestion, eat the seeds.

CONTRACEPTIVES

In India, Papua-New Guinea, and other countries, the seeds are taken as a contraceptive. For this purpose, chew 25 seeds per day well (no guarantee!). Eating the seeds or the fruit of the unripe fruit during pregnancy can lead to miscarriages. During pregnancy, women should not eat any unripe fruit or the seeds of the ripe fruit!
Some authors write that excessive consumption of the seeds can cause sterility.
Inserting a seed or ground seeds into the vagina is said to bring on menstruation (no guarantee!).

CORALS

Irritation and redness caused by the fire coral are relieved when the affected area is rubbed with very ripe or decaying fruit.

COSMETICS

The papaya cleanses the skin, digests dead skin cells, and loosens calluses. Cosmetics on a papaya basis are available from various companies. There is also soap with a papaya basis, as well as face creams, masks, lotions, and cleansing lotion (see *The Papaya in Beauty Care* on page 149).

CROUP

Remedies containing papain are available for croup.

DIABETES

Remedies containing papain help in the processing of fats and proteins, making them an excellent healing medication for those suffering from diabetes. Two tablets can be taken after meals. However, this therapy should be carried out under the supervision of a physician knowledgeable about this approach. In the Bahamas, people drink a tea from the decoction of papaya seeds for this purpose.

DIARRHEA
Green papaya or digestive remedies containing papain have proved to be useful against diarrhea (even in children). Since many children die of causes related to diarrhea in Third World countries and this natural, inexpensive remedy without side effects grows like a weed there, it should be used more often.

The Indians of Central America eat a piece of papaya with some salt several times a day against diarrhea. If you don't have any papaya, you can also drink a tea from the fruit and roots of blackberries, as the Canadian Indians do.

DIETING
See *REDUCING WEIGHT*.

DIGESTION
In all the countries where papayas are grown, the fruit is served at breakfast as a digestant to prevent or heal constipation and digestive problems. In all parts of the plant there are powerful substances that stimulate digestion. The effect of papain is not influenced by the different levels of acid or alkaline equilibrium in the digestive, as is the case for pepsin and trypsin. Papain also helps in disturbances of fat digestion (Also see *Papaya as a Digestive Aid* on page 91).

DIGESTIVE PROBLEMS
Remedies containing papain are used to support the digestion of protein, starch, and fat. Older people, who produce increasingly less hydrochloric acids and enzymes, particularly profit from digestive remedies containing papain. Papain digests 200 to 300 times its own weight in protein!

Even the juice of the green papaya, tea from the leaves, or chewing the seeds helps to alleviate all digestive disturbances such as flatulence or constipation within a short time. This approach can also help animals! A friend's dog was cured of its persistent constipation by eating half a ripe papaya every day. (Also see *Intestinal Health* on page 87 and *Papaya as a Digestive Aid* on page 91.)

DIURETIC
The ripe fruit of the papaya is recommended as a diuretic remedy.

DYSENTERY
In the tropics, the papaya is eaten as a preventive treatment against dysentery. The seeds and leaves of the fruit have also been successfully used against amebic dysentery.

DYSPEPSIA
Dyspepsia is a functional disorder of the enzyme production and output in the intestine that causes long lasting pains in the upper abdominal area. The papaya, particularly those that are not yet ripe, and remedies containing papain support digestion in a manner similar to enzyme substitution.

EAR PROBLEMS
When people have difficulty hearing, it is often due to blockage of the Eustachian tubes, which connect the middle ear with the nose. When this is blocked for a longer time, the middle ear fills with fluid. Recommendation: Drink large quantities of hot herb tea and to let a papaya enzyme tablet dissolve in your mouth four times a day.

Many pilots and stewardesses take enzyme tablets in order to keep their ears open. As a flight passenger you should carry this remedy with you and suck on a tablet four times a day.

ECZEMA
Tropical native peoples have used the milk juice of the green papaya to treat eczema for centuries. The afflicted skin area can be painted with latex juice or juice compresses can be made. An alternative is an ointment containing papain which should be included in every home first-aid kit. It also helps against itching, neurodermatitis, and dry skin areas, as well as against herpes, warts, and shingles.

ELEPHANTIASIS
In India, elephantiasis is treated by placing mashed papaya leaves on the afflicted area.

EMBOLISM
See *THROMBOSIS*.

ENZYMES

Enzymes are biocatalysts, which make life possible in the first place. They are destroyed at temperatures above 104 degrees Fahrenheit. Since enzyme preparations from plants or enzyme mixtures are dependent upon coenzymes in the form of other vital components like vitamins, minerals, and trace elements, we should basically eat raw fruit, salads, and vegetables every day. The more raw foods (organically grown, whenever possible), the better. Experts recommend that at least 30 to 50 percent of our food be eaten as raw fruits and vegetables.

Papaya enzymes like papain, chymopapain, and papayalysozym are present in the milk juice of unripe fruit at a much higher concentration than in the ripe fruit. The reason for this is that the ripening thin skin of the papaya defends itself against attacking insects with these enzymes. These "killer enzymes" benefit our bodies in digesting protein, fighting parasites, compensating for a shortage of digestive enzymes, healing wounds, and even preventing all kinds of viral infections and malignant tumors.

It is astonishing that many of these wide-ranging indications for enzyme therapy are so little known. Enzyme preparations are reliable and effective, yet they can be taken in higher doses for longer periods of time without side effects. (Also see *Enzymes and Enzyme Preparations* on page 55). It's best to find a physician or healing practitioner versed in this approach. As preventive treatment, you can also use enzymes in adequate concentrations in your food (see above) or without a prescription from the natural foods store or pharmacy.

If you are interested in more information on enzymes, you can obtain *12 Points on Natural Green Papaya Powder* discussing a number of the papaya's health effects (among others, the ability of arginine to hinder the growth of cancer) from "**Enzymes International**", Inc., Dr. Wittman Ray. See *Resources* on page 207.

If you would like to send me reports about your experiences in eating papayas, your own experiments, or experiences with papaya products, I sincerely encourage you to do so. When I have enough material and new knowledge, I plan a subsequent volume to this book. I look forward to receiving information about papayas from all over the world!

FATIGUE SYNDROME, CHRONIC (CFS)
See *CHRONIC FATIGUE SYNDROME.*

FLATULENCE
Papaya generally supports digestive weaknesses and helps avoid flatulence. Once gas has formed in the intestine, papaya makes it easier to release it. Flatulence is always a sign of a non-physiological digestive process (see also *DIGESTION* and the *Intestinal Health* on page 87).

If you wish to switch to a healthy diet of raw fruits and vegetables but have problems with flatulence at the beginning, you should fast for a few days or begin with freshly squeezed juices and slowly increase the "dose" of raw food. In the long run, raw foods are more easily digested than cooked, fried, and baked things. This especially applies to fruit since it hardly requires any digestive power!

FLU
See *COLDS, FLU.*

FRECKLES
Freckles, dark spots, and skin injuries arising from solar radiation disappear after application of ointments based on papaya, papaya face packs (see *The Papaya in Beauty Care* on page 149), or applying the ripe papaya's fruit pulp.

FUNGI (*CANDIDA ALBICANS* AND OTHERS)
A ten-percent solution of papaya juice has a good effect against yeast fungi (*Candida albicans*), which are probably the most familiar and damaging fungi. Similar results have also been attained against other types: *Candida guillierinondii* and *Candida tropicalis* (see *Papaya Combats Fungal Disease* on page 116). In addition to *Candida albicans*, there are many other yeast and mold fungi capable of inhabiting the human body and causing numerous complaints.

Strengthening the healthy intestinal flora, removing the waste substances in the intestine, and re-establishing the acid-alkali equilibrium through papain can eliminate the breeding ground for the fungi.

GAS
See *FLATULENCE*.

GASTRIC ULCER
Green papaya or remedies containing papain help prevent gastric ulcers from developing. In India, the seeds, which contain antibacterial substances, have long been eaten as a remedy against gastritis. We can also use enzyme preparations to replace pepsin and heal infections, which tend toward cancerous degeneration.

GASTRITIS
Since papain decomposes protein quickly and inhibits infection, remedies containing papain, combination enzyme preparations, and the green fruit or the seeds of the ripe fruit support gastritis therapy. Vitamin C is also important in the prevention and therapy of gastritis, and papaya contains large amounts of this vitamin. In contrast to other fruits containing vitamin C, it is well tolerated as a result of its low fruit-acid content.

GLANDS
Papayas have an exceptional effect on our endocrine gland system and help us to become healthy and stay healthy, as well as attaining ripe old age in full possession of our physical and mental powers. According to Dr. Normal Walker, this fruit has a very good effect on the thymus gland, ovaries, liver, kidneys (see *KIDNEYS*), pineal gland (see *PINEAL GLAND*), and follicles. More information can be found at the end of *Papaya Juice—A Health Cocktail* on page 59.

GLUTEN INTOLERANCE (CELIAC DISEASE)
People suffering from the celiac disease have intolerance to the gluten in wheat and other types of grains. This results in a nutritional deficiency, diarrhea, or growth disorders. Papain has proved to be successful against this illness. Patients who have eaten food without gluten for six months but still suffer from the symptoms are given an enzyme medication containing papain with every meal. After four weeks, the symptoms disappeared and did not occur again when they changed back to a normal diet.

HEART

Papaya strengthens the heart and circulatory system because active ingredients make the blood thinner, dissolve deposits in the arteries and thereby alleviate the stress on the heart. In the long run, this reduces high blood pressure (see *Papaya—Help for the Heart!* on page 114).

HEART DISEASES

A dosage of 0.2 grams of hot-water papaya extract per person has an activity-reducing effect on the human heart. Papain is also employed for "decompensated heart disease" (cardiac insufficiency). Inflammations and decay processes in the transverse colon can also adversely affect the heart function. Even here, the papaya can be helpful in the form of the entire fruit, as juice, or as a digestant containing papain. (also see *HEART*).

HEMORRHOIDS

In African countries like Ghana, the root of the papaya plant has been used against hemorrhoids since time immemorial.

HERPES

Natives of Central and South America, as well as people in India, have been using the milk juice (containing papain) from the unripe papaya for hundreds of years against all types of skin problems including herpes. For herpes simplex, there are enzyme ointments containing papain available. A simultaneous internal enzyme therapy is also recommended since the enzymes attack viruses and shorten the healing process. This lengthens the time span until the next recurrence. A herpes outbreak indicates a weak defense system, so the diet should include as much enzyme-containing raw fruits and vegetables as possible, in addition to sports, reduction of stress, and relaxation.

The herpes B virus causes the experts much greater concern. This virus is transmitted through sexual contact and leads to infections that easily become chronic; it may even become a major contributing factor toward the development of cancer of the uterus. It is being referred to as a new venereal disease of epidemic proportions. Up until now, there has been no reliable medication against this illness.

Several studies at university clinics have shown that a three-month enzyme treatment with ointments and internal administration of enzyme remedies has proved to have a healing quotient of up to 80 percent. In every case, there has at least been a distinct improvement. Both sexual partners must undergo such a treatment in order to prevent new infections.

HYDROCHLORIC ACID, DEFICIENCY OF

Many individuals, particularly older people, suffer from a deficiency of hydrochloric acid and enzymes. This creates problems in digesting protein. However, the active digestive stomach enzyme pepsin requires an acidic environment to function. This digestive weakness may result in pressure over the stomach, chronic anemia, and, in the worst case, to cancerous degeneration. Eating papaya with protein-rich meals or taking an enzyme remedy containing papain (after eating) can balance this deficit.

IMMUNE SYSTEM

The papaya strengthens the immune system so that the defensive mechanism can once again function efficiently. This is a result of the high concentration of vitamin C, the decomposition of proteometabolic products, the cleansing of the intestinal villi (see *Intestinal Health* on page 87), and acceleration of the metabolism and elimination functions. A strong defensive mechanism requires the presence of sufficient enzymes to kill viruses. Enzyme-rich fruits like the papaya help rebuild our supply of enzymes. At the same time, the papaya also delivers the necessary coenzymes in the form of vitamins, trace elements, and minerals (see *What's in the Papaya?* on page 46).

During the "cold season," many physicians recommend taking enzyme preparations as a preventive treatment to strengthen the body's defenses.

INFLAMMATION

Papain, the enzyme contained in the papaya, inhibits inflammation. It has a beneficial effect against infections, swellings, and edemas. To support healing, the traditional medicine of India and Native Americans placed slices of fruit and ground seeds on the infected skin.

Today, we can apply ointments containing papain and enzyme preparations. (Also see *GASTRITIS* and *Papaya against Inflammation* on page 1157 and *Papaya—Help for Colds and Flu* on page 113).

INJURIES

When there are injuries, the green papaya helps in particular. Mashed fruit pulp, including the skin of a green papaya, or papaya leaves can be laid on a wound as a compress. Walker reports that after applying a papaya poultice to a finger, which had been seriously crushed by a machine, he could use it in a normal way again after three days (see *BURNS*).

For poorly healing wounds, enzyme preparations have proved to be very valuable. Enzymes clean the wound bed, support healing, and prevent scars. Moreover, they help relieve the pain.

INSECT BITES AND STINGS

American physicians recommend applying ointments containing papain to painful insect bites and stings. The Native Central and South Americans applied papaya to insect stings, all kinds of animal bites, as well as injuries caused by the fire coral. Generally, the milk juice of the unripe fruit is used (see *The Papaya in the Native Central and South American Plant Therapy* on page 133). I always keep an enzyme-containing ointment like "Papaya Ointment" with me, which also helps for injuries, sprains, and sunburn.

INTESTINAL FLORA

Papaya rebuilds the beneficial intestinal flora (also see *Intestinal Health* on page 87) and functions in an antibacterial manner. Healthy intestinal flora is necessary for good digestion and optimal distribution of nutrients to the cells.

LARYNGEAL DIPHTHERIA (TRUE CROUP)

In India, the larynx is painted with the milk juice of the papaya (see *The Papaya in the Folk Medicine of India* on page 137).

LIBIDO, POTENCY

According to Oberbeil, eating papayas strengthens the libido for both men and women. The abundance of enzymes in the papaya provides optimal stimulation for the sexual glands. All inner organs and glands have better circulation and remain active up into old age when given the proper, enzyme-rich nutrition.

We can also see exotic fruits such as papayas, mangos, and pineapples as a natural remedy in the battle against impotency and frigidity. Research has also shown that people who remain sexually active when older, stay healthier, are more content, and live longer than those whose sexual life has fallen by the wayside.

LIVER

Many people suffering from a liver disease cannot tolerate fruit. Papaya is an exception to this situation. It is "a wonderful healing food for liver disorders and a valuable help, even in the most sensitive cases" (A. Vogel). The ripe fruit can therefore be recommended for sluggish liver activity.

You can eat the fruit fresh or take remedies containing papain such as "Papayaforce" or other remedies based on papaya-enzymes. Walker recommends the juice of the green and ripe papaya to strengthen the liver function (see the end of *Papaya Juice—A Health Cocktail* on page 59).

The people of India cook the young leaves of the papaya as a vegetable to cleanse the liver. Enzyme preparations should be taken as support in the case of hepatitis (inflammation of the liver).

MALARIA

In the folk medicine of India, the young leaves of the papaya are cooked as vegetables and eaten against malaria.

MASSAGE

In India, oil based on papaya, which you can easily prepare yourself, is used as a popular massage oil (see recipe in *The Papaya in the Folk Medicine of India* on page 137).

MENSTRUAL COMPLAINTS

Women in countries where the papaya originated eat the seeds when they have menstrual complaints.

METABOLISM

The papaya—preferably the green but also the ripe fruit, as well as the seeds of the ripe fruit and the leaves—stimulates the metabolism, removes waste from the intestine (and other areas), and helps detoxify the liver.

MISCARRIAGE

Women from Native Central and South American tribes and Polynesian are said to eat the unripe papaya or seeds in order to cause a miscarriage (see *The Papaya in Native Central and South American Plant Therapy* on page 133 ff). Similar Information comes from India and Papua-New Guinea. For this reason, pregnant women should avoid the seeds of the ripe fruit and the fruit pulp of the unripe papaya (also see CONTRACEPTION).

MULTIPLE SCLEROSIS (MS)

MS patients should take remedies containing papain on a regular basis because it eliminates the toxic effect of wheat gluten. Combined enzyme preparations have a beneficial effect (see *Enzyme Preparations* on page 55). They can also lead to healing in many cases, which can only seldom be expected from orthodox MS therapy. There appears to be a correlation between viruses and multiple scleroses, which explains the success of enzyme therapy. Particularly good results have been obtained with the "Dr. Evers Diet." Authentic Reiki has helped many MS patients and is used in the Paracelsus Clinic on the German island of Helgoland.

MUSCLE TENSION

In the folk medicine of India, an oil is made on the basis of the papaya (for recipe, see *The Papaya in the Folk Medicine of India* on page 137). This is rubbed into the skin for joint and muscle pain. It is also used by women experiencing muscle tension after a birth or against muscle paralysis after a stroke.

NUTRITION

The papaya greatly enriches our diet. It contains more vitamin C than an orange or kiwi, a large amount of beta carotene (the precursor of vitamin A), much vitamin D, and some B vitamins, as well as numerous minerals and so-called "bioactive substances." Some experts consider the latter to be a cancer-preventing remedy (see section on *CANCER*).

In addition, papaya is a strongly alkali-forming food (see *Help against Acidosis* on page 77) and removes waste deposits in the body. It is extremely low in calories. Because of its high enzyme content, it breaks down proteins, fats, and carbohydrates quickly. This makes it is easier to lose weight, even without reducing the amount of food eaten. Papain also helps to keep the cholesterol level low.

The papaya is easy to digest and therefore also recommended as a baby food.

OPERATIONS

Taking an enzyme preparation a few days before and after an operation has a definite beneficial effect: it supports the healing of wounds and edemas (water accumulation), thrombosis (blood clot), and inflammations (see corresponding keyword and chapter) occur less frequently.

PANCREAS

When there is a disorder of the pancreas, protein digestion is complicated and an unpleasant feeling of fullness results after meals containing protein. If you eat papaya or, for example "Papayasan"—made from the leaves and the juice of unripe papaya—after protein-containing food, this feeling of fullness often disappears after a few minutes. Together with kelp preparations (potassium iodine), "Papayasan" has also proved useful against pancreatic fatty stools and pancreatitis. Since it is well tolerated, papaya is used, especially in geriatrics, in the form of enzyme combinations.

PARASITES

Intestinal parasites are inactivated by the active ingredients carpaine and papain, which are found in green papaya and the seeds of the ripe fruit (also see *WORMS*).

PHLEBITIS

See *VARICOSE VEINS*.

PINEAL GLAND

In his book *The Natural Way to Vibrant Health,* Dr. Norman W. Walker writes that ripe papayas are one of the most valuable forms of nutrition for the pineal gland when eaten together with fresh raw carrot juice: This mixture is one of the healthiest for the human body. The pineal gland is considered to be the receptive organ of cosmic energy and is connected with the adrenal glands and the reproductive organs. The thyroid gland converts the energy so that it is available for the human body. Qualities such as staying power, energy, and strength are said to be dependent upon the proper functioning of the pineal gland. (Information about the papaya with regard to other glands can be found at the end of *Papaya Juice: A Health Cocktail* on page 59).

The Aborigines use papaya flowers in order to come into contact with their higher self (also see *A Papaya Meditation* on page 156).

PROTEIN SUPPLY AND DIGESTION

The Germans are number one worldwide when it comes to consuming animal proteins! Today, the average German eats 220 pounds of meat and sausage per year. In 1900, the average German ate only 30 pounds of meat. In addition, large quantities of milk products are consumed. Such excess consumption of protein leads to protein deposits in the vessels, to hyperacidity (see *ACIDOSIS* and *Help against Acidosis* on page 77), and to protein-storage diseases. After the age of 35, the lack of enzymes leads to a miserable digestion of protein. To remedy this situation, a "papaya treatment" is recommended: Eat one papaya every day for a week. I recommend continuing this cure indefinitely!

For intestinal cleansing, you can also chew about one tablespoon of papaya seeds on an empty stomach in the morning. It would naturally be even better, with respect to cancer prevention, to cut the amount of animal proteins in half and only eat meat once a week. It has been established that vegans, who have a vegetarian diet without eggs and milk products, do not suffer from a lack of protein. Instead, they are healthier than the so-called lacto-vegetarians (more information in *Cancer—Causes and Alternatives* on page 95).

PURIFICATION

Papain has a purifying effect on the entire organism. It removes waste deposits, detoxifies, and cleanses. Nutritional waste is thoroughly digested and eliminated by papain. In addition, the digestive enzyme removes toxins from the inner organs. A raw food diet and fast cures once a year are recommended to keep the body clean.

REDUCING WEIGHT

Because of its wealth of enzymes, the papaya helps stimulate your digestion. Weight reduction is facilitated when proteins, carbohydrates, and fats are broken down more effectively and quickly. If you eat the seeds with the ripe fruit, your digestion will be activated in addition to losing weight without side effects because papaya doesn't irritate the intestine. Instead, it protects and cleanses it.

The papaya became known for its weight-reducing qualities through the "Beverly Hills Diet," which recommends tropical fruits because of their abundance of enzymes.

REJUVENATION

The papaya is said to have a rejuvenating effect. There isn't a more powerful "intestinal cleaner" for our body! Dr. B. Lytton Bernard has a health center in Guadalajara, Mexico. He says that the cleansing effect of the papaya goes far beyond the digestive tract, also extending to all tissue (also see *Intestinal Health* on page 87 and *Help against Acidosis* on page 77).

Vasco da Gama supposedly called the papaya "the golden tree of eternal youth" and the Chinese have always viewed it as "the fruit of a long life." Dr. Norman W. Walker also assumed that papayas exert a rejuvenating influence on our organs by harmonizing and stimulating almost all of the glands (more details in the chapter on *Papaya Juice: A Health Cocktail* on page 59).

RHEUMATISM

Rheumatic complaints have been treated with great success (internally and externally as ointment) by papain and other plant and animal enzymes. The advantage is that they break down the infection physiologically, dissolving the dispersed immune complexes so that they cannot become new sites of infection. At the same time, they do not suppress the body's own immune system the way most rheumatism medications do. In addition, they have no side effects when taken for extended periods at high doses.

Dr. Klaus Hoffmann recommends papaya expressly to rheumatism patients in his German-language book on rheumatism: The lack of fruit acids is beneficial for the stomach and they seldom cause allergies. I would like to add that the special alkali-forming effect of the papaya is very important for rheumatism patients, who all suffer from hyperacidity!

RICKETS

The people of India rub the lower extremities with a papaya-root extract with alcohol added to treat rickets.

SEXUALLY TRANSMITTED DISEASES

The boiled root of the papaya is one component of a prescription against sexually transmitted diseases. In India, a decoction is cooked from the bark and taken in small liqueur glasses against syphilis. In East Africa, an infusion of the root is used against syphilis.

Papain also helps in enzyme preparations against the "new venereal disease" of type B herpes because enzymes are "virus killers" (see *HERPES*).

SHINGLES

I don't know if the natives of Central and South America also use the papaya for shingles. However, today enzyme remedies containing papain are used very successfully against this illness (and, as a preventive treatment, when someone in the family has chicken pox). Since shingles can cause complications (including meningitis, scarring, blindness, and cancer), Gerhard Leibold considers it malpractice if the therapist does not prescribe an enzyme ointment and a remedy consisting of enzyme mixtures for internal use against this viral disease. Sometimes complications such as nerve pain, which can last for months, disappear a few hours after the enzyme therapy begins. A complete absence of symptoms can be achieved in a week.

If your physician isn't informed about the success of enzyme therapy, you can turn to a naturopath or take enzyme medication, which is available without a prescription in every pharmacy, on your own with no fear of side effects.

SKIN

For centuries, the people in the countries where papayas grow have been using the milk juice of the green papaya for skin-care purposes in order to cleanse the skin and make it softer. There are also lines of cosmetics on a papaya basis (also see *COSMETICS* and *Papaya in Beauty Care* on page 149).

I have had good results in treating neurodermatitis caused by a food allergy with an ointment containing papain: The itching stopped and the skin regenerated.

SORE THROAT

In the Philippines, people eat the green papaya to heal a sore throat in order to digest dead tissue and mucous. Healthy tissue is not affected. If green papayas are not available, you can slowly chew the seeds of the ripe fruit or a few pieces of ripe pineapple. The latter contains an enzyme that has a similar effect.

Enzyme preparations also help against colds and sore throats (see *COLDS, FLU*): Allow one papaya enzyme tablet to dissolve slowly in your mouth four times a day. When used for tonsillitis, the same treatment decreases swelling of the tonsils and increases the effectiveness of antibiotics.

SPORT INJURIES

In combination with other enzymes, papaya remedies are used by athletes as a preventive treatment, as well as for the treatment of internal and external sport injuries.

SPRAINS

For sprains and bruises, the Indians of Mexico apply the following poultice: Mix one tablespoon of dried papaya seeds and pumpkin seeds with one cup of water, dry the mixture in the sun (alternative: in the oven at low heat), and apply the paste to the affected area (see *MUSCLE TENSION*).

STOMACH

Papain helps to balance disturbances of the gastro-intestinal secretion, which is particularly advantageous for older people, who produce less hydrochloric acid and digestive enzymes with increasing age. In combination with plant substances, papaya is used as in enzyme mixtures against digestive and stomach disturbances. The folk medicine of India recommends the ripe fruit against stomach disorders and digestive disturbances in general.

SUNBURN

In Australia and New Zealand, there are ointments based on papayas that are very effective against sunburn. If you eat lots of fruits and vegetables containing much beta-carotene, like papayas, mangoes, broccoli, wild herbs and algae, it is unlikely to get a sunburn at all. This is my experience. Another possibility is to eat as much raw food as possible.

TEETH

There is a tooth powder based on the papaya, "Papaya Tooth Powder." This powder not only cleans the teeth but also helps with problems such as gingivitis (inflammation of the gums) or bleeding from the gums.

As a result of its very high vitamin-C content, the ripe papaya (fruit pulp and seeds) can be used to prevent and heal bleeding gums and periodontosis (see *What's in the Papaya?* on page 46). Solutions containing papain are also added to cleaning solutions for false teeth. When teeth are extracted, the use of enzyme remedies before and after the surgery has proved to be helpful. Pain is reduced and the wound heals better without swelling, and the development of edema is also prevented.

THROMBOSIS, EMBOLISM

In general, eating papaya or other enzymes containing papain keeps the blood thin and therefore prevents thrombosis. Arteriosclerosis is an important risk factor for thrombosis because changes in the vessel walls and the thickness of the blood favor its development (also see *HEART*). Thrombosis becomes extremely dangerous when a clot of blood breaks loose and blocks an artery. Enzymes are also capable of dissolving blood clots and preventing such "micro-thrombosis" from covering themselves with a fibrin net, which protects them from the body's own defense system.

TIREDNESS, CHRONIC

Chronic tiredness often is related to an attack of fungi or parasites, which strain the organism by releasing toxins. Here as well, the papaya helps as a vermicide and antifungal medication (also see corresponding chapter). If you don't want to take an enzyme remedy, you can chew papaya seeds in the morning on an empty stomach. Or mix granulate with water, eat green papaya, or make a habit of using papaya pepper on your food (see *Recipes for the Kitchen* on page 162). Papaya is an alternative to grapefruit seed extract, which tastes bitter and is usually refused by children for this reason. (Also see *CHRONIC FATIGUE SYNDROME.*) Many people feel an instant lift-up after eating papayas and don't need coffee in the morning or in the afternoon. Try it out!

TRAVEL FIRST-AID KIT

In his remedy book, Vogel recommends that one take a digestive medication made from papayas with you on all trips to the tropics or sub-tropics: Take two tablets after every meal in order to protect yourself from digestive disorders and worm infestation.

Many Indians chew a papaya leaf the size of a half-dollar before every meal to prevent infections and parasite infestation. On my travels, I take a combined enzyme remedy with me so that I can support injuries and accelerate the healing process in case of possible inflammations, infections, or injuries. For external use, I take along an ointment containing papain, which can be obtained from natural food stores or a pharmacy without a prescription. "Nature's First Law" offers health trips to papaya lands such as Florida and Hawaii.

TUBERCULOSIS

Carpaine, which is found in the green papayas and leaves of the plant, has an anti-bacterial effect and has been used successfully against tuberculosis.

VARICOSE VEINS, PHLEBITIS

Papain has been used successfully together with other enzymes in the treatment of varicose veins and other vein disorders. Enzyme preparations and consumption of papaya on a regular basis help thin the congested blood in varicose veins. Enzyme ointments should also be applied externally. Symptoms of phlebitis clear up considerably faster, reducing dangerous complications such as thrombosis and embolism (also see *THROMBOSIS*).

An accompanying sport program (see *Sport Is Suicide?—Movement is Life!* on page 20) and learning Authentic Reiki are also recommended to improve circulation in the legs, as well as a diet rich in alkaline and raw fruits and vegetables. (See *ACIDOSIS* and *Help against Acidosis* on page 77.)

VENEREAL DISEASE

See *SEXUALLY TRANSMITTED DISEASES*.

WARTS

For centuries, the natives of the papaya countries have rubbed the juice into warts. Even today, papain is still applied externally to warts to remove dead tissue.

A firm papaya can be cut or peeled and the white, sticky juice applied without dilution to the wart. Do not apply undiluted to healthy skin or mucous membrane and keep away from the eyes! If this should happen accidentally, rinse with a large amount of cold water. If rubbing the warts with milk juice doesn't do the job, the folk medicine of India recommends binding a piece of the tree bark over the wart for 24 hours to make it disappear. However, applying an enzyme ointment usually is adequate. In persistent cases, an enzyme preparation can also be taken internally.

WEIGHT LOSS

The papaya is invaluable for people who want to lose weight. It contains few calories and accelerates both the metabolism and digestion (see also *REDUCING WEIGHT*).

WORMS

Inhabitants of tropical islands use the white juice of the green papaya and the seeds of the ripe fruit against worms: as therapy and preventive treatment for human beings and animals. As an alternative to the latex juice (dilute 1:1 with water), an additional recipe is used in the folk medicine of India: Boil the roots with garlic in one cup of water, let it thicken to half the volume, and take half of this amount twice a day with milk.

In dogs infested with Ascaris lumbricoides, a dosage of 2/3 ounce of papaya juice per pound of body weight has been determined to kill this maw-worm. For worm infestation of human beings and animals, grinding of the black papaya seeds into powder is recommended. Dissolve a teaspoon of the powder in warm water and drink every three hours. Papaya-seed granulate can also be taken. An alternative: papaya tea from leaves. For further information, see *Papaya Gets Rid of Worms* on page 122.

WOUNDS

Remedies containing papain are used to dissolve "false flesh." The natives of Central and South America have always used papaya to cover putrefying wounds.

There are several ointments like Papaya Ointment with a papain basis available for healing gangrenous wounds. Remedies containing papain help without attacking healthy tissue (also see *BURNS*). Festering and badly healing wounds can be treated successfully with freshly squeezed papaya leaves. Vogel reports that even Bagdad boils—"*ulcera tropica*"—respond to this method. An alternative: enzyme ointments containing papain.

Additional Uses for the Papaya

BEER

Papain is used to cleanse beer, except in countries like Germany where the purity regulations prohibit additives.

MEAT TENDERIZER

In the West Indies and other tropical islands, there is a century-old practice of wrapping meat in papaya leaves to make it tender.

Another recipe for this purpose is rubbing tough meat with slices of green papaya and cooking it together with a meal containing meat. Today, papain is widely used as a meat tenderizer, especially in the USA.

In order to avoid deceiving the consumer, the use of papain as a meat tenderizer is prohibited in Germany: After treatment with papain, meat that was as hard as leather becomes as tender as that from a young animal. If the papain is used for too long, the meat decays. In the USA, animals are even sprayed shortly before slaughtering them to make the meat more tender. Knowing this, should motivate you to reduce or drop your meat consumption.

PLANTS

In his German-language book on enzyme therapy, Kurt Allgeier reports that protein-splitting enzymes can also be successfully used against the viral infections of plants. When tobacco and bean plants were sprayed with enzymes or had them injected into their stems, the infection was immediately arrested. The leaves that had not yet been attacked remained healthy. When the enzyme was applied to healthy plants as a preventive treatment, 60 percent of the plants remained completely healthy and the rest suffered distinctly less damage than untreated plants.

I have had good experience in using this approach against mites: I added one teaspoon of ground, dried papaya seeds to the spray water. After spraying three times within one week, the plants were free of mites and had a good recovery.

Enzyme therapy proved successful for plants and is used today especially in raising valuable flowers such as orchids and on tobacco plantations.

TANNING

Papain is used in tanning to make leather and fur soft, as well as to manufacture wool and silk that don't shrink.

Appendix

A Papaya A Day

A papaya a day keeps the doctor a-way. Take two or three and you will see: You feel healthy and fine, and you'll start to shine! Life gets happy as could be, life gets happy as could be!

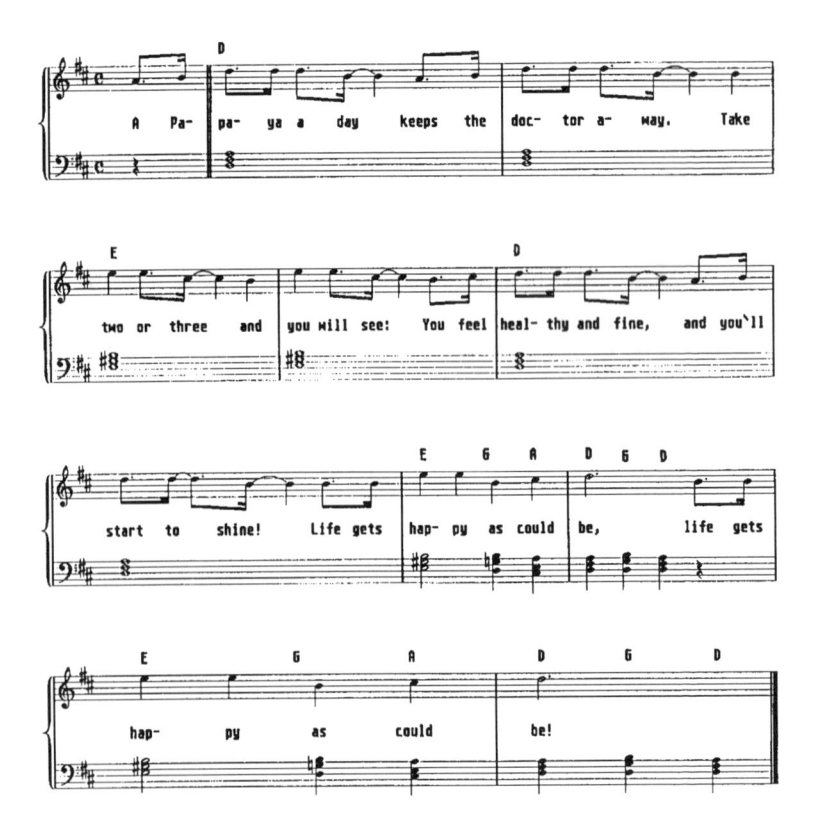

A Papaya a day keeps the doctor away. Take two or three and you will see: You feel healthy and fine, and you'll start to shine! Life gets happy as could be, life gets happy as could be!

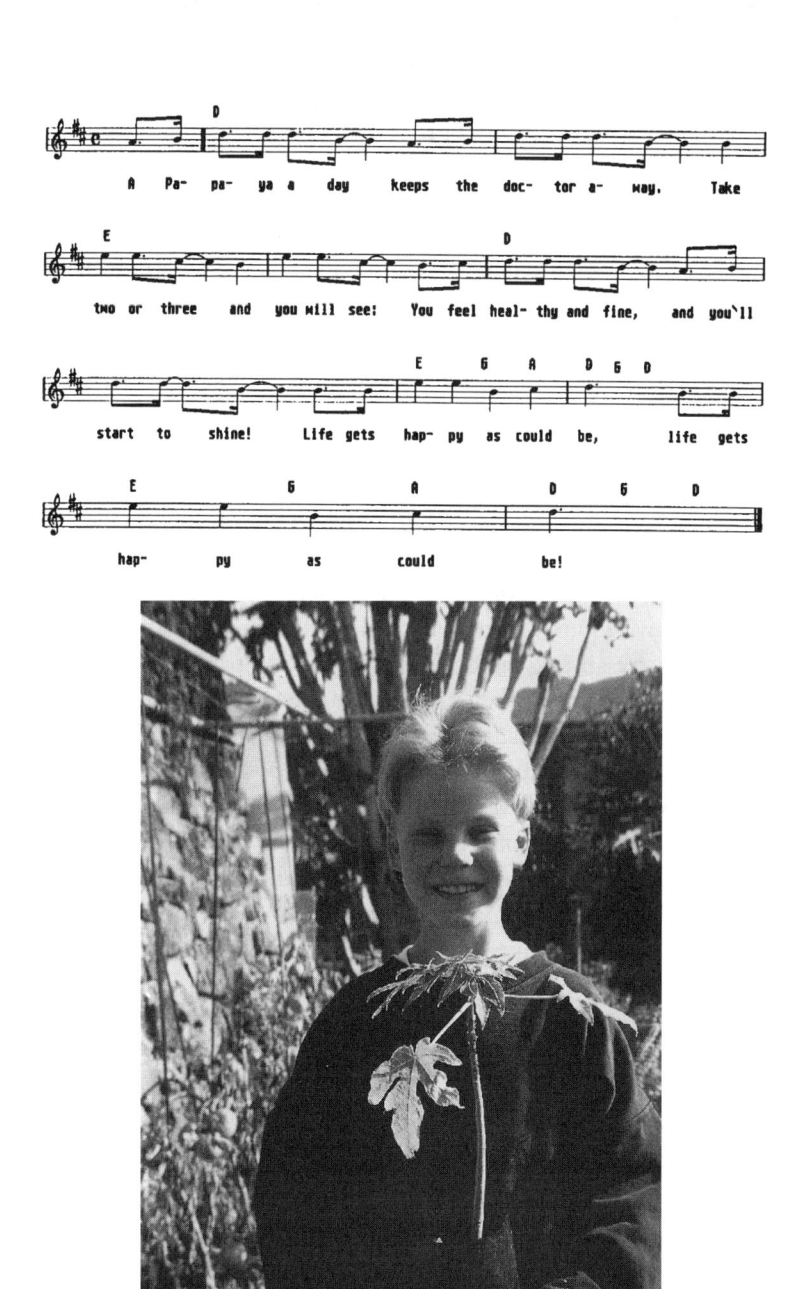

Michael, 9-year-old, with a small papaya plant, which will be replanted soon

Papaya Products

Many readers of this book will probably look for papayas in natural food stores, supermarkets, and produce stores during the next weeks or months in order to make the recommended dishes, dry the fruit, or prepare the enzyme-rich papaya pepper themselves (see *Recipes for the Kitchen* on page 160).

Some firms offer organically dried papaya, and others will send fresh organic papayas per express mail. (Additional supply sources can be found by searching the Internet under the keyword of "papaya products".)

Granulate, powder, and enzyme bars are available from Papaya John in Hawaii (see corresponding chapter) and from "Papaya Power". Teas, enzyme preparations, and nutritional supplements containing papaya can be found at most natural food stores. Perhaps you will decide to try an enzyme ointment containing papain, an enzyme remedy, or papain powder. These can also be purchased at the most natural food stores, health food stores, or pharmacies.

(**Caution**: Be careful not to get the papain powder in your eyes! If you do, wash out the eyes immediately with cold water. The same applies to liquid papain or the milk juice of the unripe fruit.)

There are also many cosmetic lines, including the "Green Papaya Enzyme Products" (see *Papaya in Beauty Care* on page 149) manufactured by the firm Beauty Naturally and a skin care line by Kneipp Cure distributed by Papaya Power.

In the USA, there are many other products based on papayas: from chewing gum to face creams, digestant pills, cleaning solutions, contact-lens cleaners, meat tenderizers, and many more. Papain is used in 80 percent of American beers, and even Coca-Cola is made with it. If you should be allergic to papayas, which occurs very rarely, you will have problems in the USA: It's almost impossible not to come in contact with papaya!

In Australia, there is a tincture based on papaya for healing small wounds, a tea from papaya leaves, and various other products that are mostly cosmetic in nature.

Call for International Cooperation

I hope you are now inspired by the many possibilities that papaya offers for improving our health—and there certainly is much more to discover!

Perhaps you have pets and want to use papaya to improve their health. Perhaps stockbreeders, farmers, animal keepers, veterinarians, and healing practitioners who work with animals will want to try treating their animals with these safe enzymes.

With respect to plants, there are certainly many possibilities as well. The German firm Merck, which manufactures papain, has reported success in using it as a plant-protecting and pest-control agent. However, it has stopped its research in this direction because of the related costs. Wolf, the founder of enzyme therapy, carried out successful experiments with enzymes in the garden. If you eat papayas and dry the seeds, you can make a liquid containing papain and use it against lice and mites on your indoor plants and balcony plants (also see *PLANTS* in the *Additional Uses for the Papaya* section on page 198).

If you should find an interesting new use for papaya and gather your own wealth of experiences, please don't just keep this information to yourself! For this purpose, I have established the "Papaya Forum" to collect information and possible areas for use. As soon as this information is supported by similar experiences, scientific studies, or reports from the field of ethno-medicine, I would like to publish it for the benefit of all and post it on the Internet.

Please send interesting experiences, observations, and knowledge related to the benefits of the papaya, as well as how people in other countries use it, to:

PAPAYA FORUM
c/o Theo Hodapp
Holbeinstr. 26
22607 Hamburg
Germany
e-mail: Basim@Barbara-Simonsohn.de

If possible, please send the information written in English, German, Dutch, or French.

Together with a doctor specialized in ethno-medicine, I plan to make a video program on the papaya. If you wish to contribute film material, you are heartily invited to do so. Please contact the above address for this purpose.

One major request: Please don't ask me questions such as "Does papaya or a specific enzyme product have an effect on this type of symptom?" Address such questions to your healing practitioner, physician, or directly to the manufacturer of these products. For chronic problems, you should always consult a specialist. Don't engage in self-medication with enzyme preparations, papaya, or papaya products in the place of a personal consultation! Your problems may have a serious organic cause and, in individual cases, these products may possibly not be effective enough.

Acknowledgments

At this point I would like to specially thank Theo Hodapp, who surfed in the Internet, searched through libraries, and lovingly cared for our two children while they had to be very considerate of their mother and her work. Thanks also to three-year-old Freya, who has protected me from visitors with "psst, mother is working!" and Michael, nine years of age, who inspired me time and again with his curiosity and dry humor.

Thanks to Dr. Katharina Boeddeker, who took the time to correct my manuscript even during the hectic last phase of the book and greatly motivated me with her praise and enthusiasm!

Thanks also to my parents who raised me to question everything, and who have "infected" me with their love of plants.

Thanks also to my grandfather, who turned 104 years old in August of 1999 and showed me through his example that it is possible to keep our mental and physical powers at this ripe, old age.

Thanks to Helmut Wandmaker, my "old, young" friend who brought the literature of "Natural Hygiene" to Germany. Through his books and the uncompromising example of his lifestyle, he has helped many people regain their health and joy in life.

Thanks also to Franz Konz for his courage and his persistence as living proof that cancer does not have to mean infirmity when we radically transform our lives and let ourselves fall into the arms of nature.

Thanks to Baldur Springmann, an untiring fighter for organic farming and gardening, for his support and the opportunity of spending a year learning from him and through him at the Springe Farm.

And thanks to Anna Schroeder, who didn't always have an easy time with me during my apprenticeship at the *Schulungszentrum fuer naturgemaessen Land- und Gartenbau in Hohenbuchen* ("School Center for Natural Farming and Gardening in Hohenbuchen"), from whom I have learned a great deal about life of the soil and organic soil care.

Thanks to Halima Neumann, who inspired me time and again with her enthusiasm about the healing power of the papaya, for being another living example that cancer can be conquered. As a result, she has given many people new hope of healing, even from this disease.

Thanks to Stephen Arlin and David Wolfe from San Diego, two raw food enthusiasts and best-selling authors. By their example, they show that radiant health is our true birthright. It only waits to be rediscovered and embraced at every moment by the decisions we make in everyday life.

Thanks to Winfried Veldung, who gathered information for me about ethno-medical uses of the papaya in the voodoo culture, in China, and in Vietnam.

Thanks to Astara Kim Hill from Hawaii, for her extensive research about the papaya as a healing plant of the kahunas in Hawaii.

Thanks to all my friends in the USA, the Canary Islands, Australia, and Germany who have helped me to put together the information.

Thanks to Bodo J. Baginski, who inspired me to write a book on the topic of "papaya," and thanks to Monika Juenemann, my publisher, who was once again willing to take a courageous, trailblazing step in publishing it.

From the bottom of my heart, I would like to also thank all my friends and readers who are enthusiastic about the papaya and natural ways of becoming healthy, who use this knowledge and share it with others: You are making a contribution toward a healthier and more natural lifestyle, as well as healing the earth and our children and their children.

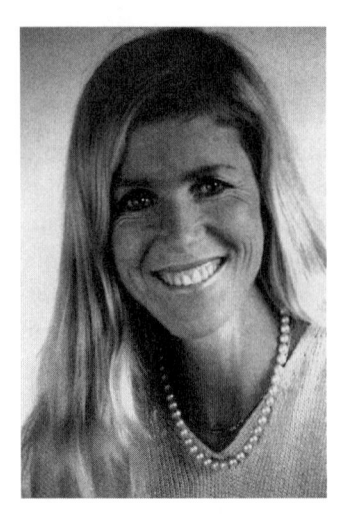

The Author

Barbara Simonsohn was born in Germany on January 29, 1954. After graduating from the *Gymnasium* (college-prep high school), she studied sociology at Hamburg University and concluded her studies as a political scientist. She worked as a public relations manager for an organization that sponsors exchange programs for young people before she decided to learn about organic farming and gardening.

For ten consecutive years, she was at Findhorn Community in Scotland for holidays, where she not only worked in the garden but also learned the holistic methods of healing. For one-and-a-half years, she studied at the biodynamic organic farm *Hof Springe*, then at the school for natural farming and gardening in Hohenbuchen.

At the Hamburg adult education program, she taught the first environmental courses on environmental topics, elevated plant beds, and organic gardening. During this time, Barbara Simonsohn wrote articles on alternative lifestyles for *Szene Hamburg* and the *Hamburger Abendblatt* newspapers.

When she was in her mid-twenties, Barbara Simonsohn met Dr. Renate Collier, a Mayr therapist and naturopathic physician. She underwent an intestinal-cleansing treatment with her, organized the first seminars with her, and trained to teach seminars on acidosis.

Since this time, Barbara Simonsohn has been primarily interested in healthy nutrition and has changed her own diet. She first became a vegetarian, and then switched to eating only whole foods and raw vegan foods according to the theories of "Natural Hygiene."

In 1984, Barbara Simonsohn completed her education as a teacher of Authentic Reiki with Dr. Barbara Ray in the USA. Since then, she has held seminars on learning this simple technique for stress relief, deep relaxation, activation of self-healing powers, and personal development in the German-language region, the USA, and the Canary Islands.

Her son Michael was born in 1988 and her daughter Freya was born in 1994. She lives with her children in a home with a large garden in Hamburg, Germany. Here she not only has flowers but also organically grown vegetables and fruit, including a few mountain papaya trees.

When Barbara Simonsohn became inspired about the topic of this book, she dedicated the largest part of her time to international research and studying the effects of the papaya on herself. Enthused by her results, she reduced her time spent holding seminars and lectures to write about her collected knowledge and experiences. This book represents the results of this research.

Resources

The Reader's Service Department of the publishing company maintains an up-to-date Internet list with producers and distributors of the papaya products mentioned in this book, as well as important contact addresses for:
- Information on papaya
- Papaya products
- Juicers
- Health centers
- Organic fruit, fresh and dried
- Papaya seeds
- Papaya videos
- Magazines
- Cancer clinics with a natural, holistic approach
- Raw food restaurants
- Seminars
- Retreats

This list is updated on a regular basis.

Look under **www.windpferd.com** click on the American flag (International English Version), click on the button service-addresses, scroll for the title *Healing Power of Papaya* and then click for the complete list of papaya resources.

Notes

1. Elke Bolz: *Super Teint*, p. 125.
2. Henning Allmer, Psychologist: "Biologie der Erholung" in *Focus* 24/1997.
3. Quoted by Dr. Friederich. W. Dittmar: *Enzyme, Aktivstoffe für Frauen*, p. 116.
4. Norman Walker: *Colon Health*.
5. Vasant Lad: *Ayurveda—Science of Self-Healing*, p. 38.
6. Ibid, p. 69.
7. Norman Walker: *Colon Health*
8. T.C. Frey: *Program for Dynamic Health: An Introduction to Natural Hygene*.
9. Shalila Sharamon and Bodo J. Baginski: *The Healing Power of Grapefruit Seed*, p. 41.
10. Harvey and Marilyn Diamond: *Fit for Life*.
11. Ibid.
12. Ibid.
13. Harish Johari: *The Healing Cuisine: India's Art of Ayurvedic Cooking*.
14. Ibid.
15. Helmut Wandmaker: *Willst du gesund sein, vergiß den Kochtopf!*, p. 117.
16. Burger, Guy-Claude: *Die Rohkosttherapie*, p. 257.
17. Ibid, p. 277 and 278.
18. Ibid, p. 44.
19. Ibid, p. 44.
20. Ibid, p. 45.
21. Quoted by Chester French: *Papaya—The Melon of Health*, p. 10. French refers to a handwritten text from the Vatican Library, discovered and translated by the American Charles Upson Clark and published by the Smithsonian Institute in Washington, D.C. on September 1, 1942.
22. Hans Peter Rusch: *Bodenfruchtbarkeit*, p. 221.
23. Max Gerson: *A Cancer Therapy: Results of 50 Cases and the Cure of Advanced Cancer*.
24. Ibid.
25. Ibid.
26. Hans Peter Rusch: *Bodenfruchtbarkeit*, p 129.
27. Ibid, p.235.
28. Alwin Seifert: *Gaertnern, Ackern ohne Gift*, p. 210.
29. Ingeborg Münzing-Rulf: *Kursbuch gesunde Ernaehrung*, p. 192.
30. Dr. Edward Howell: *Enzyme Nutrition*.
31. Ibid.
32. Klaus Oberbeil and Dr. Christiane Lentz: *Obst und Gemuese als Medizin*, p. 56.
33. Quoted according to C. and M. Raschka: *Ueber die Urspruenge der Krankenheilung…*," p. 948.

34. Dr. Max Wolf: *Enzyme Therapy.*
35. Helmut Wandmaker: *Willst du gesund sein, vergiß den Kochtopf!,* p. 177.
36. Norman Walker: *Raw Vegetable Juices.*
37. Ibid.
38. Ibid.
39. Ibid.
40. Klaus Oberbeil and Dr. Christiane Lentz: *Obst und Gemuese als Medizin,* p. 15.
41. Gerhard Leibold: *Enzyme,* p. 72.
42. Norman Walker: *The Vegetarian Guide to Diet and Salad.*
43. Patrick Geryl: *Peak Performance Foods.*
44. Quoted according to Helmut Wandmaker: *Willst du gesund sein, vergiß den Kochtopf!,* p. 172.
45. Ibid, p. 171.
46. Dr. Edwin Flatto: *Super Potency at Any Age.*
47. Patrick Geryl: *Peak Performance Foods.*
48. Ibid.
49. Ibid.
50. Ibid.
51. Dr. Christiane May-Ropers and David. Schweitzer: *Nie wieder sauer,* p. 24.
52. Ibid., p. 109.
53. Ibid,, p. 109.
54. Karl O. Glaesel: *Heilung ohne Wunder und Nebenwirkungen. Gesundheit biologisch gesteuert,* p. 170.
55. Ibid., p. 101 and p. 166.
56. Hermann Aihara: *Acid & Alkaline.*
57. Halima Neumann: *Stop Krebs, MS, AIDS. Eine neue Ganzheitsmethode,* p. 159.
58. Wolfgang Spiller: *Dein Darm, Wurzel der Lebenskraft,* p. 32.
59. Edward Bach: *Heal Thyself,* about 1920.
60. Wolfgang Spiller: *Dein Darm, Wurzel der Lebenskraft,* p. 16.
61. Norman Walker: *Colon Health.*
62. Dr. John Henry Kellog in: *Physical Culture,* July 1940.
63. Dr. David Chowry Muther (private doctor of Mahatma Gandhi) in: *Nature's Path,* November 1935.
64. Dr. K. R. Krogmann: "Was ist Papaya" in *Volksgesundheit,* no. 8, 1971.
65. Dr. Hans Nieper: *Revolution in Medizin und Gesundheit,* p. 95.
66. Dr. K. Renner and Dr. J. H. Cantler: *Ernährung und Krebs.*
67. Ibid, p. 95.
68. John H. Tilden, *Toxemia Explained.*
69. Carrington Hereward: *Vitality, Fasting and Nutrition.*

70 Louis Kuhne: *The New Science of Healing*, p. 32-33, quoted by ibid.
71 Ross Horne: *Improving on Pritkin—You Can Do Better!*
72 Helmut Wandmaker: *Willst du gesund sein, vergiß den Kochtopf!*, p. 171.
73 Ibid., p. 323.
74 Ross Horne: *Improving on Pritkin—You Can Do Better!*
75 Ibid.
76 Quoted by Helmut Wandmaker: *Willst du gesund sein, vergiß den Kochtopf!*, p. 22.
77 A. T. Hovannessian: *Raw-Eating* (out of print).
78 Hans Nieper: *Revolution in Medizin und Gesundheit*, p. 151.
79 Harvey and Marilyn Diamond: *Fit for Life*.
80 Max Gerson: A Cancer Therapy: *Results of 50 Cases and the Cure of Advanced Cancer*.
81 Norman Walker: *Raw Vegetable Juices*.
82 Kurt Allgeier: *Die Enzymtherapie*, p. 85.
83 Gerhard Leibold: *Enzyme*, p. 80.
84 Kurt Allgeier: *Die Enzymtherapie*, p. 109.
85 Hermann Geesing: *Die beste Waffe des Koerpers: Enzyme*, p. 116.
86 Halima Neumann: *Stop Krebs, MS, AIDS ...*, Preface.
87 Ibid., Preface.
88 Helmut Wandmaker: *Willst du gesund sein, vergiß den Kochtopf!*, p. 255
89 Wolfgang Spiller: "Neurodermatitis" in Hans Baumgardt: *Ursache und Heilung von Allergien*, p. 79.
90 Gerhard Leibold: *Enzyme*, p. 47.
91 Helmut Wandmaker: *Willst du gesund sein, vergiß den Kochtopf!*, p. 139.
92 Gerhard Leibold: *Enzyme*, p. 68.
93 Ibid., p. 61.
94 Helga Vollmer: *Enzyme fuer die Frau*, p. 125.
95 Wolfgang Spiller: *Dein Darm, Wurzel der Lebenskraft*, p. 55.
96 Ulla Kinon: *Mycosen, die (un)heimliche Krankheit*.
97 Ibid., p. 150
98 A. Vogel: *Die Leber als Regulator der Gesundheit*, p. 100.
99 Dr. Klaus-Ulrich Hoffman: *Rheuma heilt man anders*, p. 60.
100 Ravi Roy and Carola Lage-Roy: *Homeopathische Ratgeber Reisen*, p. 19.
101 Quoted by Christian Ratsch: *Indianische Heilkraeuter*, p. 197.
102 Ibid. p. 197f.
103 Vasant Lad: *Ayurveda—Science of Self-Healing*, p. 29.
104 Friederich-W. Dittmar: *Enzyme, Aktivstoffe für Frauen*, p. 138.
105 Gerhard Madaus: *Lehrbuch der biologischen Heilmittel*, volume I, p. 845.

Bibliography

Aihara, Hermann. *Acid & Alkaline.* Oroville, CA: George Ohsawa Macrobiotic Foundation, 1986.

Airola, Paavo. *How to Get Well: Dr. Airola's Handbook of Natural Healing.* Health Plus Publications, 1971.

Airola, Paavo. *How to Keep Slim, Healthy, and Young with Juice Fasting.* Health Plus Publications, 1971.

Aivanhov, Omraam Mikhael. *Yoga of Nutrition.* Proseveta, 1991.

Allgeier, Kurt. *Die Enzymtherapie.* Dusseldorf, Germany: Econ. Verlag, 1978.

Allmer, Henning. "Biology der Erholung" in: *Focus* 24, 1997.

Arlin, Stephen. *Raw Power! Building Strength and Muscle Naturally.* Maul Brothers Publishing, San Diego, CA 1998.

Arvigo, Rosita and Balick, Michael. *Rainforest Remedies: 100 Healing Herbs of Belize.* Twin Lakes, WI: Lotus Press Publications, 1993.

Bach, Edward. *Heal Thyself.* London: Daniel, 1946.

Banarjee, Pradas, Dr. *Materia Medica of Indian Drugs, vol. 1, 1977, key word: Carica Papaya.* Howrah 711101: Shiva & Co. Medical Publishers.

Barnard, Neal. *Eat Right, Live Longer.* New York: Harmony Books, Crown Publishers, Inc., 1995.

Berlin Woche, No. 36, 1997 "Können Melonen klettern?"

Blauer, Stephan. *The Juicing Book.* Garden City Park, New York: Avery Publishing Group Inc., 1989.

Bolz, Elke. *Super Teint.* Niedernhausen, Germany: Falken Verlag, 1995.

Branch, W. J. *The British Medical Journal* of June 16, 1906.

Bragg, Paul C. and Bragg, Patricia. *The Miracle of Fasting.* Santa Barbara, CA: Health Science, 1999.

Bragg, Paul C. and Bragg, Patricia. *The Toxicless Diet: Body Purification and Healing System.* Santa Barbara, CA: Health Science, 1997.

Brown-Jordan, Portia. *Herbal Medicine and Home Remedies. A Potpourri in Bahamian Culture.* Nassau/New Providence, Bahamas: The Nassau Guardian Printing Press, 1986.

Carper, Jean. *The Food Pharmacy—Dramatic New Evidence That Food is Your Best Medicine.* New York: Bantam Books, 1988.

Carrington, Hereward. *The History of Natural Hygiene.* Mokelhumne Hill, CA: Healthy Research, 1964.

Carrington, Hereward. *Vitality, Fasting and Nutrition.* New York: Rebman Company, 1963.

Chan, Harvey T. Jun. and Tang, Chung-Shih. "The Chemistry and Biochemistry of Papaya" in Inglett, Caratambus (editor) *Tropical Foods*, vol. I, p. 33 ff. USA: Academic Press, 1979.

Chopra, Dr. Deepak. *Perfect Health: The Complete Mind/Body Guide.* New York: Harmony Books, 1990.

Cichoke, Anthony J. *The Complete Book of Enzyme Therapy.* Avery Publishing Group, 1998.

Cichoke, Anthony J. *Enzymes & Therapy.* Connecticut: Keats Publishing Inc., 1994.

Cinque, Ralph C. *Quit for Good: How to Break a Bad Habit.* Canada: Monarch Books, 1997.

Clark-Regehr, Hulda. *The Cure of All Cancers: 100 Case Histories.* San Diego, California: ProMotion Publishing, 1993.

Clark-Regehr, Hulda. *The Cure for all Diseases.* San Diego, California: ProMotion Publishing, 1995.

Claus, Edward P. and Tyler, Varro E. *Pharmacognosy.* Philadelphia: Lea & Febiger Verlag, 1965.

Collier, Renate. *Wie neugeboren durch Darmreinigung.* Munich, Germany: Verlag Gräfe und Unzer, 1995.

Cooper, Dr. Kenneth H. *Antioxidant Revolution.* Thomas Nelson, 1997.

Cupta, Wambebe and Parsons. "Central and Cardiovascular Effects of the Alcoholic Extract of the Leaves of Carica Papaya," No. 4, p. 257-266, Swets & Zeitlinger, in: *J. Crude Drug Res.*, 28, 1990.

Diamond, Harvey. *You Can Prevent Breast Cancer.* Pro Motion Pub., 1996.

Diamond, Harvey and Marilyn. *Fit for Life.* New York: Warner Books, 1985.

Diamond, Marilyn and Schnell, Donald Burton. *Fitonics for Life.* New York, N.Y.: Avon Books, 1998.

Dinshah, Freya. *The Vegan Kitchen.* Malaga, New Jersey: American Vegan Society, 1970.

Dittrich, K. and Leitzmann, Dr. C. *Bioaktive Substanzen.* Stuttgart, Germany: Georg Thieme Verlag, 1996.

Duke, James Alan and Vasquez, Rodolfo. *Amazonian Ethnobotanical Dictionary.* Ann Harbor: CRC Press, 1994.

Flatto, Edwin. *Super Potency At Any Age.* Miami, Florida: The Plymouth Press, 1991.

Fox, Dr. Michael. *New Eden, For People, Animals, Nature.* Twin Lakes, WI: Lotus Press.

Frawley, Dr. David. *Ayurveda and the Mind.* Twin Lakes, WI: Lotus Press, 1997.

Frawley, Dr. David and Lad, Dr. Vasant. *Yoga of Herbs, Ayurvedic Guide.* Twin Lakes, WI: Lotus Press, 1986.

Frähm, David and Anne. *Healthy Habits. 20 Simple Ways to Improve Your Health.* Penguin Putnam Inc., New York, 1993.

French, Chester. *Papaya—The Melon of Health.* New York: Arco Publishing Company, 1972.

Frohn, Birgit, Uber, Heiner, and Xokonoschtletl. *Medizin der Mutter Erde, die alten Heilweisen der Indianer.* Munich, Germany: Mosaik Verlag, 1996.

Fry, T. C. *The Curse of Cooking.* Austin, Texas: Life Science, 1975.

Fry, T.C. *Program for Dynamic Health: An Introduction to Natural Hygiene.* Manchaca, Texas: Health Excellence System, 1992.

Fry, T. C. *Super Foods for Super Health.* Austin, Texas: Life Science, 1976.

Geesing, Dr. Hermann. *Die beste Waffe des Körpers: Enzyme.* Munich, Germany: F. A. Herbig Verlagsbuchhandlung, 1990.

Gelfand, M., Mavi, S., Drummond, R. B., and Ndemera, B. *The Traditional Medical Practicioner in Zimbawe: His Principles of Practice and Pharmacopoeia.* Zimbawe: Mambo Press, 1986.

Gerson, Dr. Max. *A Cancer Therapy: Results of 50 Cases and the Cure of Advanced Cancer.* Talman Co., 1997.

Glaesel, Karl O. *Heilung ohne Wunder und Nebenwirkungen. Gesundheit biologisch gesteuert.* Constance, Germany: Labor Glaesel Verlag, 1994.

Hagiwara, Yoshihide. *Green Barley Essence, the Ideal Fast Food.* Keats Publishing, Connecticut, 1985.

Hartwell, H. L. "Plants Used Against Cancer" in *Lloydia 31 (71)*, p. 108-9, 1968.

Heideklang, Christine. *Mykosen.* Munich, Germany: Droemersche Verlagsanstalt, 1995.

Heinerman, John. *Heinerman's New Encyclopedia of Fruits and Vegetables.* Prentice Hall, New Jersey, 1995.

Herrmann, Dr. Karl. "Über die Aromastoffe exotischer Obstarten—III. Papaya und andere Caricaceen, annonaceen, Kiwi, Litschee, Solanum-Arten" in: *Flüssiges Obst,* vol. 62, No. 1-2, 1995.

Herrmann, Dr. Karl. "Produkte aus exotischen Obstarten: Mango, Papaya, Guava und Avocado" in: *Guardian, Nov. 94,* p. 174-176.

Herrmann, Dr. Karl. "Über die Inhaltsstoffe und die Verwendung wichtiger exotischer Obstarten" in: *Industrielle Obst- und Gemüseverwertung,* 80, 1995, p. 7-9.

Herrmann, Dr. Karl. "Über die Inhaltsstoffe und die Verwendung wichtiger exotischer Obstarten, II. Papaya" in: *Industrielle Obst- und Gemüseverwertung,* Feb. 94, p. 34-46.

Hewitt, B. E. "*Sensitivity testing with the Chymo-FAST Test*" in *Neurochirurgia 29,* p. 154-155, Stuttgart, Germany: Georg Thieme Verlag, 1986.

Hill, Ann (Ed.). *A Visual Encyclopedia of Unconventional Medicine.* New York: Crown Publishers, 1979.

Holler, Johannes. *Iß Dich klüger. Das praktische Handbuch für die optimale Gehirnernährung.* Frankfurt, Germany: Umschau Verlag, 1997.

Horne, Ross. *Improving on Pritikin—You can do better!* Australia: HarperCollins, 1988.

Hovannessian, A T. *Raw Eating.* Teheran, Iran: Arshavir, 1967.

Howell, Dr. Edward. *Enzyme Nutrition—The Food Enzyme Concept.* Wayne, New Jersey: Avery Publishing Groups, Inc., 1985.

Howell, Dr. Edward. *Food Enzymes for Health and Longevity.* Twin Lakes, WI: Lotus Press, 1994.

Inglett, George E. and Chartambus, George. *Tropical Foods,* vol. 1. USA: Academic Press, Inc. , 1979.

Jenuwein, Heinz. *Avocado, Banana Coffee: How to Grow Useful Exotic Plants for Fun.* (Out of print)

Johari, Harish. *The Healing Cuisine: India's Art of Ayurvedic Cooking.* Rochester, Vermont: Inner Traditions International Ltd., 1994.

Juchheim, Jürgen K. and Poschet, Jutta. *Immun.* Munich, Germany: BLV Verlagsgesellschaft, 1996.

Junemann, Monika and Luetjohann, Sylvia. *Three Great Healing Herbs.* Twin Lakes, WI: Lotus Light, 1998.

Karsten, Uwe. *Die geheimen Erfolgsrezepte der Voodoo-Medizin.* Germany: Medien & Natur Verlagsgesellschaft.

Kellog, Dr. John Harry. In: *Physical Culture*. July 1940.

Kenton, Leslie and Susannah. *Raw Energy*. London: Fisteba, 1984.

Kloss, Jethro. *Back to Eden, Revised Edition*. Twin Lakes, WI: Lotus Press, 1998.

Kordich, Jay. *The Juiceman's Power of Juicing*. New York: William Morrow & Co., *1992*.

Kranz, Brigitte. *Das große Buch der Früchte*. Munich, Germany: Südwest Verlag, 1971.

Krok, Morris. *Fruit, the Food and Medicine for Man*. Natal, South Africa: Essence of Health, 1967.

Kuhne, Louis (see Carrington, Hereward and note 69)

Küthe, Gerhard and Spoehase, Hajo. "Anbau und Nutzungsmöglichkeiten von Papaya" in *Der Tropenlandwirt*, Oct. 1974, p. 129-139.

Lad, Vasant. *Ayurveda—Science of Self-Healing*. Twin Lakes, WI: Lotus Press, 1984.

Leibold, Gerhard. *Enzyme*. Niedernhausen, Germany: Falken Verlag, 1994.

Lewis, Walter H. *Medical Botany: Plants Affecting Man's Health*. London: John Wiley & Sons, 1977.

Lindner, Dr. M. "Die Papayafrucht" in: *Deutschen Apothekerzeitung*, volume 111, July 22, 1971.

List, P.H. and Hörhammer, L. *Hagers Handbuch der Pharmazeutischen Praxis*. Berlin, Germany: Springer Verlag, 1972.

Lötschert, Dr. Wilhelm and Beese, Dr. Gerhard. *Collins Guide to Tropical Plants: A Descriptive Guide to 323 Ornamental and Economic Plants*. (Out of print).

Lucas, Dr. Thomas. *The Papaw*. Brisbane, Australia: The Carter-Watson Co.

Lubeck, Walter. *Healing Power of Pau D'Arco*, translated by Christine M. Grimm. Twin Lakes, WI: Lotus Light, 1998.

MacKenzie, R.A. and Strachan, G. "Possibilities for Processing Mountain Papayas in New Zealand" in *Food Technology in New Zealand*, August 1980, No. 8, p. 13 and 19.

Maier, Christian. *Das Leuchten der Papaya*. Hamburg, Germany: Europäische Verlagsanstalt, 1996.

Markowitz, Elysa. *Warming up to Living Foods*. Book Publishing Company, Sommertown, 1998.

Markowitz, Elysa. *Living with Green Power*. Alife Books, Burnaby BC, Canada, 1997.

Mayer, H.-M. "Inzidenz und Verhütung allergischer Reaktionen nach Chemonukleolyse mit Chymopain" in: *Neurochirurgia 29*, p. 149-153, Stuttgart, Germany: Georg Thieme Verlag, 1986.

Mayr, Dr. Franz X. *Schönheit und Verdauung*. Alberschwende, Austria: Verlag Neues Leben, 1991.

Mazel, Judy. *The New Beverly Hills Diet*. Health Communications, 1996.

Meyerowitz, Steve. *Wheat Grass—Nature's Finest Medicine. The Complete Guide to Using Grasses to Revitalize Your Health*. Sproutman Publications, Massachusetts, 1998.

Miller, John J. "Papaya" in *Northwest Technocrat*, vol. IX, No. 105, 1945.

Miller, Richard Alan. *The Magical and Ritual Use of Aphrodisiacs*. Rochester, Vermont: Inner Traditions International Ltd., 1993.

Moneret-Vautrin, Felmann, Kanny, Baumann, Roland, and Pere. "Incidence and Risk Factors for Latent Sensitization to Chymopapain: Predictive Skin-Prick Tests in 700 Candidates for Chemonucleolysis" in *Clinical and Experimental Allergy*, volume 24, p. 471-476, 1994.

Morgan, Marlo. *Mutant Message Down Under*. New York: HarperCollins Publ., Inc., 1995.

Müller, Harald. *Institute of Nutritional Physiology*: "Determination of the Carotenoid Content in Selected Vegetables and Fruits by HPLC and Photodiode Array Detection," p. 88-94. Berlin, Germany: Springer Verlag, 1997.

Murray, Michael T. *The Complete Book of Juicing: Your Delicious Guide to Youthful Vitality*. Rockland, CA: Prima Publications, 1997.

Muther, Dr. David Chowry, in *Nature's Path*. London, Nov. 1935.

Neale, Donald Walsh. *Conversations with God. Book 1,2,3*. Hampton Roads Publishing Company, Charlottesville, 1996-1998.

Neumann, Halima. *Stop Krebs, MS, AIDS, Eine neue Ganzheitsmethode*. Starnberg, Germany: Fürhoff Verlag, 1997.

O'Hare, Paul. *Growing Papaws in South Queensland*. Queensland, Australia: Department of Primary Industries, 1995.

Polunin, Miriam. *Healing Foods*. London: Dorling Kindersley, 1972.

Randolph, Dr. Theron G. and Moss, Dr. Ralph W. *An Alternative Approach to Allergies: The New Field of Clinical Ecology Unravels Environmental Causes*. New York: HarperCollins, 1990.

Ratsch, Christian. *Plants of Love: Aphrodisiacs in Myth, History, and the Present*. Ten Speed Press, 1997.

Rauch, Erich. *Diagnostics According to F.X. Mayr: Criteria of Good, Marginal, and Ill Health*. Medicina Biologica, 1983.

Richard, David. *My Whole Food ABC's*. Vital Health Publishing, Bloomingdale, 1997.

Richard, David, Byers, Dorie. *Taste Life! The Organic Choice*. Vital Health Publishing, Bloomingdale, 1998.

Robbins, John. *Diet for a New America: How Your Food Choices Affect Your Happiness and the Future of Life on Earth*. USA: H. J. Kramer, 1998.

Rochlitz, Steven. *Advanced Human Ecology and Energy Balancing Sciences: Toward a Science of Healing*, vol. II. Sedona, AZ: Human Ecology Balancing Sciences, 1989.

Rochlitz, Dr. Steven. *Allergies and Candida with the Physicist's Rapid Solution*. Sedona, AZ: Human Ecology Balancing Sciences, 1997.

Rusch, Hans Peter. *Bodenfruchtbarkeit*. Heidelberg, Germany: Karl F. Haug Verlag, 1991.

Santillo, Humbart. *Food Enzymes: Missing Link to Radiant Health*. Twin Lakes, WI: Lotus Press, 1993.

Schaller, Dr. Christian Tal. *Mes secrèts de Santé-Soleil*. Chène-Bourg, Switzerland: Editions Vivez Soleil, 1992.

Secretaria de Agricultura. *Frutas de Colombia para el Mundo*. Columbia: Medellin, 1991.

Seibold, Ronald L. *Cereal Grass, What's in It for You!* Wilderness Community Education Foundation, Lawrance, Kansas, 1990.

Sharamon, Shalila and Baginski, Bodo J. *The Healing Power of Grapefruit Seed*. Twin Lakes, WI: Lotus Light, 1996.

Sharma, Dr. Hari. *Awakening Nature's Healing Intelligence*. Twin Lakes, WI: Lotus Press.

Sharma, Dr. Hari. *Freedom from Disease: How to Control Free Radicals*. Twin Lakes, WI: Lotus Press, 1993.

Shelton, Dr. Herbert M. *Fasting Can Save Your Life.* USA: American Natural Hygiene Society, 1978

Shelton, Dr. Herbert M. *Food Combining Made Easy.* USA: Willow Publishing, 1940.

Shelton, Dr. Herbert M. *Health for All.* USA: Kessinger Publ. Co., 1997.

Shelton, Dr. Herbert M. *The History and Principles of Natural Hygiene.* USA: Kessinger Publ. Co., 1997.

Shelton, Dr. Herbert M. *Superior Nutrition.* San Antonio, TX: Dr. Shelton's Health School, 1961.

Simonsohn, Barbara. *Stevia—sündhaft süß und urgesund.* Aitrang, Germany: Windpferd, 1999.

Simonsohn, Barbara. *Die sagenhafte Heilkraft der Ananas.* Aitrang, Germany: Windpferd, 1998.

Simonsohn, Barbara. *Gerstengrassaft—Verjüngungselixier und naturgesunder Power-Drink.* Aitrang, Germany: Windpferd, 1999.

Simonsohn, Barbara. *Die Fünf Tibeter mit Kindern.* Wessobrunn, Germany: Integral Verlag, 1995.

Snowdon, Anna L. *A Colour Atlas of Post-Harvest,* vol. 1. London, England: Wolfe Publishing Ltd., 1990.

Soleil, Docteur. *Apprendre à se nourir.* Chêne-Bourg, Switzerland: Editions vivez Soleil, 1993.

Steinegger, Ernst and Hänsel, Rudolf. *Pharmakognosie.* Berlin, Germany: Springer, 1992.

Storl, Wolf-Dieter. *Pflanzendevas—Die Göttin und ihre Pflanzenengel.* Aarau, Switzerland: AT, 1997.

Svoboda, Robert. *Prakruti: Your Ayurvedic Constitution.* Twin Lakes, WI: Lotus Press, 1989.

Tarabilda, Edward F. *Ayurveda Revolutionized: Integrating Ancient and Modern Ayurveda.* Twin Lakes, WI: Lotus Press, 1998.

Tang, Chung-Shih. "Macracyclic Piperdine and Piperideine Alkaloid in Carica Papaya" in Inglett, Charatambus: *Tropical Foods,* vol. I., p. 55ff, USA: Academic Press Inc., 1979.

Teuscher, Eberhard. *Pharmazeutische Biologie.* Germany: Friedr. Vieweg Verlag, 1989.

Tierra, Dr. Michael. *Planetary Herbology.* Twin Lakes, WI: Lotus Press, 1987.

Tietze, Harald. *Papaya (Pawpaw), The Medicine Tree.* Bermagui South, NSW, Australia: Harald W. Tietze Publishing, 1997.

Tietze, Harald. *Kombucha: The Miracle Fungus.* Australia: Three Books, 1996.

Tilden, Dr. John H. *Toxemia Explained: The True Interpretation of the Cause of Disease.* USA: Kessinger Pub., 1997.

Tiwari, Bri. Maya and Benedict, Dirk. *Ayurveda Secrets of Healing.* Twin Lakes, WI: Lotus Press, 1995.

Upson, Charles (see French, Chester and Note 24)

Vogel, A. *A. Vogels Gesundheitsratgeber.* Teufen, Switerland: Verlag A. Vogel, Teufen, Switzerland 1997.

Vogel, A. *Der kleine Doktor.* Munich, Germany: Wilhelm Heyne Verlag, 1997.

Vogel, A. Health Guide through Southern Countries. Subtropical, Tropical and Desert Zones. Verlag A. Vogel, Teufen, Switzerland, 1987.

Vogel, A. *Die Leber als Regulator der Gesundheit.* Teufen, Switzerland: Verlag A. Vogel, Teufen, Switzerland 1985.

Vogel, A. *Krebs—Schicksal oder Zivilisationskrankheit?* Teufen, Switzerland: Verlag A. Vogel, Teufen, Switzerland 1987.

Vollmer, Helga. *Enzyme für die Frau.* Berlin, Germany: Verlag Sport und Gesundheit, 1995.

Wagner, Dr. Hildebert. *Pharmazeutische Biologie—Drogen und ihre Inhaltsstoffe.* Stuttgart—New York: Gustav Fischer Verlag, 1993.

Walker, Dr. Norman W. *Become Younger.* Prescott, AZ: Norwalk Press, 1976.

Walker, Dr. Norman W. *Colon Health.* Prescott, AZ: Norwalk Press, 1979.

Walker, Dr. Norman W. *The Natural Way to Vibrant Health.* Prescott, AZ: Norwalk Press, 1995.

Walker, Dr. Norman W. *Pure and Simple Natural Weight Control.* Prescott, AZ: Norwalk Press, 1981.

Walker, Dr. Norman W. *Raw Vegetable Juices.* Prescott, AZ: Norwalk Press.

Walker, Dr. Norman W. *The Vegetarian Guide to Diet and Salad.* Prescott, AZ: Norwalk Press, 1971.

Walker, Dr. Norman W. *Water Can Undermine Your Health.* Prescott, AZ: Norwalk Press, 1974.

Walker, Dr. Norman W. and Langer, Manfred G. *Zurück aufs Land zur Selbstversorgung.* Ritterhude, Germany: Waldhausen Verlag, 1995.

Wandmaker, Helmut. *Rohkost statt Feuerkost.* Munich, Germany: Wilhelm Goldmann Verlag, 1996.

Wandmaker, Helmut. *Willst du gesund sein, vergiß den Kochtopf!* Munich, Germany: Wilhelm Goldmann Verlag, 1992.

Webb, Edwin C. *Enzyme Nomenclature.* San Diego—New York—Boston—London—Sydney—Tokyo—Toronto: Academic Press, 1992.

Weiss, R. F. und Fintelmann, V. *Herbal Medicine.* Medicina Biologica, 1988.

Wendth, Lothar. *Gesund Werden durch Abbau von Eiweißüberschüssen.* Germany: Ragnar Berg.

Wigmore, Ann. *Be Your Own Doctor. A Positive Guide to Natural Living.* Avery Publishing Group, Wayne, New Jersey, 1982.

Wigmore, Ann. *The Hyppocrates Diet and Health Programm.* Avery Publishing Group, Inc., Wayne, New Jersey, 1983.

Wigmore, Ann. *Why Suffer? How Overcome Illness and Pain Naturally.* Hippocrates Health Institute, 1985.

Wolfe, David. *The Sunfood Diet Success System. 36 Lessons in Health Transformation.* Maul Brothers Publishing, San Diego, CA 1999.

Wrba, Heinrich. *Systemische Enzymtherapie.* Munich, Germany: MMV Medizin Verlag, 1996.

Wrba, Heinrich and Pecher, Otto. *Wirkstoffe der Zukunft. Mit der Enzymtherapie das Immunsystem stärken. Entzündungen, Rheuma, Viruserkrankungen, Krebs.* Vienna—Zurich—Munich: Orac Verlag, 1995.

Index

A

Acid-alkali equilibrium 19, 50, 56, 77, 79–85, 90, 92, 120, 183, 188, 191, 198
Acid-forming foods 77, 83
Acidosis 1, 15, 24, 28, 31, 65, 77, 78–84, 117, 126, 160, 167, 173, 190, 191, 192, 197, 208
Additives 39, 97, 111, 198. *Also see* Preservatives
Adrenal glands 65, 66, 173, 191
Aging 21, 26, 44, 49, 56, 57, 61, 66, 69, 74, 96, 127, 149, 159, 183, 192
AIDS 11, 57, 99, 173, 211, 212, 217
Alcohol 14, 15, 33, 51, 52, 77, 83, 90, 97, 119, 137, 142, 160, 174, 193, 214
Algae 18, 70, 82, 85, 88, 89, 107, 195
Alkaline 78, 79, 80, 82–85, 91, 102, 176, 181, 198, 212, 213
Allergies 1, 11, 14, 24, 49, 57, 78, 80, 90, 91, 111, 112, 117, 118, 124, 129, 174, 193, 217
Amebic dysentery 142, 174, 181
Amino acid 27, 92, 93
Amino acids 92
Antibiotics 57, 116, 119, 194
Appetite 32, 50, 123, 124, 137, 175
Arginine 70, 93, 130, 182
Arteriosclerosis 56, 80, 114, 115, 167, 175, 195
Arthritic pain 134, 137
Arthritis 23, 28, 56, 93, 99, 112, 127, 175
Arthrosis 173, 175
Ascarids 122, 123, 125, 138
Asthma 98, 111–113, 118, 134, 137, 142, 145, 167, 176
Authentic Reiki 15, 18, 26, 83, 113, 121, 156, 189, 197, 208
Autointoxication 89, 92
Ayurveda 24, 25, 139, 140, 210, 212, 214, 216, 218, 219

B

Baby food 90, 190
Backaches 23, 126, 127, 129, 176
Bacteria, putrefying 83
Basic. *See* Alkaline
Beauty 14, 19, 23, 51, 60, 69, 149–150, 158, 159, 161, 179, 183, 194, 202
Beer 39, 51, 174, 198, 202
Beriberi 49, 136, 142
Beta carotene 62, 72, 100, 149, 161, 189

Bilharziasis 123, 130
Bioactive substances 15, 27, 190
Birth 88, 117, 143, 152, 154, 176, 189, 205
Birth control 176. *Also see* Contraceptives
Bladder 79, 107, 116, 130, 131, 134, 136, 140, 142, 145
Bliss 29, 140
Blood pressure 11, 21, 50, 61, 65, 66, 81, 93, 98, 106, 114, 133, 136, 167, 176, 185
Bones 50, 80, 89, 126
Bowel movement 55, 89, 112, 138
Breast 38, 40, 56, 93, 100, 111, 141, 146, 214
Breast cancer 100, 146, 214
Bronchitis 116, 118, 136, 137, 142, 145, 153, 167, 176, 178
Bruises 48, 134, 141, 177, 194
Burns 56, 103, 134, 137, 177, 187, 198

C

Calcium 47, 48, 50, 66, 80, 92, 115, 171
Cancer 11, 12, 14, 16, 21, 39, 42, 46–49, 52, 55–57, 59, 62, 69, 70, 78–80, 85, 89, 93, 95, 96, 98–112, 116, 120, 124, 136, 137, 140, 143, 145–149, 154, 159, 160, 167, 168–174, 177, 182, 184, 185, 186, 190, 191, 193, 205, 210, 212, 214, 215
Candida 117–119, 121, 124, 177, 183, 217
Capacity 41, 49, 79, 113
Capillary circulation 81
Carbohydrates 27, 47, 61, 81, 82, 97, 100, 117, 119–124, 190, 192
Cardiac arrest. *See* Heart attack
Carpaine 46, 82, 106, 115, 130, 136, 140, 142, 176, 190, 196
Carrot juice 63, 170, 191
Cell structure 78
Cellulite 149, 167–170, 178
CFS. *See* Chronic Fatigue Syndrome
Cheese 58, 82, 83, 91, 160, 164, 167, 178
Chemonucleolysis 104, 126–130, 167, 176, 217
Chemotherapy 106, 172
Children 15, 22, 26, 30, 49, 55, 57, 60, 62, 74, 78, 80, 91, 111, 113, 117, 118, 120, 123, 124–126, 133, 137, 138, 145, 146,

161, 164, 174, 180, 196, 204, 206, 208
Chlorella 85
Cholesterol 61, 72, 97, 115, 190
Cholesterol level 61, 190
Chronic fatigue syndrome 178, 183, 196
Cigarettes 14, 17, 142
Circulation 21, 23, 42, 54, 81, 89, 174, 176, 188, 197
Colds 14, 48, 78, 84, 99, 112–115, 138, 178, 183, 187, 194
Colitis 113, 178
Concentration, lack of 48, 118
Constipation 11, 23, 50, 89, 93, 119, 133, 140, 141, 146, 179, 180
Contraceptives 136, 176, 179
Coral 179, 187
Cosmetics 128, 149–152, 179, 194
Coughs 142, 153
Course of treatment 56, 84
Cow's milk. *See* Milk
Croup 175, 179, 187
Croup, true. *See* Laryngeal diphtheria

D

Dandruff 153
Deep relaxation 83, 208
Defensive powers 112
Degeneration 47, 70, 108, 113, 184, 186
Deposits, waste 89, 90, 92, 121, 140, 167, 169, 190, 192. *Also see* Deposits, waste
Detoxification 60, 171
Diabetes 59, 81, 93, 100, 173, 179
Diarrhea 89, 113, 119, 134, 136, 140, 141, 146, 171, 178–181, 184
Diet 14–17, 18, 27–30, 53, 62–65, 69, 70–73, 77–81, 84, 85, 87, 88, 90, 91, 93, 95, 97, 98, 100–102, 107, 108, 111–116, 117, 119–126, 130, 139, 140, 149, 157, 178, 183–186, 189, 191, 192, 197, 208, 211, 213, 216, 217, 219, 220
Digestion 28, 47, 49, 51, 55, 60, 90, 92, 93, 94, 101, 134, 138, 139, 161, 167, 168, 176, 179, 180, 181, 187, 190–193, 197
Digestive disorder 176
Digestive Enzyme 94
Digestive enzyme 192
Digestive weakness 186
Dried fruit. *See* Fruit dried
Drugs 51, 53, 62, 70, 131, 138, 213
Dysentery 87, 141, 142, 181
Dyspepsia 140, 181

E

Ears 128, 181

Eggs 15, 90, 93, 119, 122, 125, 167, 171, 191
Elevated plant bed. *See* Plant bed, elevated
Elimination 14, 29, 55, 60, 65, 93, 96, 139, 186
Enemas 103
Energy 12, 13, 15, 23, 28, 29, 51, 60, 60–64, 71, 72, 84, 87, 101, 117, 118, 123, 139, 140, 154, 156, 191, 216, 217
Environment 25, 43, 77–81, 87, 91, 92, 98, 117, 120, 139, 149, 186
Environmental poisons 117
Enzyme 35, 38, 51–58, 67, 70, 71, 75, 82, 83, 88–92, 94, 103–106, 107, 108, 112, 114–116, 121, 125, 128, 136, 137, 140, 149, 150, 151, 154–158, 159, 161, 163, 170, 173–179, 181, 182, 184–191, 192–199, 202–205, 210–216, 216, 219
Enzyme deficiency 52, 53, 140
Ethno-Medicine 55, 75, 116, 132, 177
Ethno-medicine 11, 132, 203, 204
Exercise 14, 15, 21–23, 53, 58, 64, 70, 97, 102, 113, 126, 127, 176, 178
Exhaustion 14, 79, 84, 96

F

Farming 205, 207
Fasting 29, 60, 61, 84, 121, 131, 156, 211, 213, 218
Fatigue 119, 178
Fatigue Syndrome, Chronic. *See* Chronic fatigue syndrome
Fats 61, 81, 90, 97, 100, 168, 179, 190, 192
Fermentation 82, 88
Fertility 38, 41
Fertility, soil. *See* Soil fertility
Fertilizer 39, 45, 61, 98, 111, 160
Fever 62, 113, 114, 131, 137, 138, 142
Fiber 29, 97, 121, 127, 169
Fish 82, 90, 123, 167, 168
Five Tibetan Rites. *See* Tibetan Rites, Five
Flatulence 92, 93, 118, 119, 121, 140, 153, 180, 183, 184
Flora, intestinal 11, 53, 87, 88, 90, 92, 112, 119, 120, 136, 183, 187
Flour, white 77, 111
Flu 99, 113, 114, 138, 178, 187
Foods, sun 71, 72
Foods, whole 84, 98, 208
Freckles 137, 150, 152, 183
Fruit 10, 11, 15, 16, 18, 19, 27, 28–40, 42, 43, 45–48, 53, 54, 59–63, 63, 68, 69, 71–74, 77, 78, 82, 85, 90, 92–95, 98, 99, 101, 103, 106, 107, 108, 110,

219

114, 120, 122, 124, 130–134, 136–138, 140–145, 147, 148, 151–154, 156, 157, 161–170, 173, 174, 176–180, 180, 181, 182–190, 192–196, 197, 202, 208, 216
Fruit, Dried 161
Fungus 109, 117–120, 121, 147, 168, 218

G

Garden 18, 21, 23, 30, 36, 38, 44, 59, 89, 108, 149, 156, 203, 207, 208, 213
Gardening, organic 207
Garlic 70, 89, 120, 138, 145, 163, 165, 170, 171, 198
Gas. *See* Flatulence
Gastric ulcer 184
Gastritis 93, 184, 187
Germs 41, 46, 87, 116
Glands 22, 23, 53, 64–67, 70, 71, 73, 149, 169, 173, 184, 188, 191, 192
Glucose 28, 48
Gout 82, 138
Grains 87, 90, 150, 184

H

Healing 1, 11, 12, 17, 18, 26, 28, 48, 49, 53, 54, 56, 57, 59, 60, 62, 63, 64, 65, 82, 83, 93, 94, 96, 101, 104, 107–111, 113, 115–118, 124, 130, 132, 133, 136, 139, 143, 146–151, 149, 154, 158–161, 167, 171, 173, 177, 179, 182, 185–191, 196, 198, 202–210, 210, 212, 213–216, 218, 219
Healing Power 1, 26, 124, 210, 216, 218
Healing power 54, 65, 110, 148, 149, 159, 205
Healing practitioner 17, 64, 117, 182, 204
Health insurance 17, 18, 127, 129
Heart 5, 14, 21, 24, 44, 46, 48–52, 54, 59, 60, 69, 71, 78, 85, 93, 95, 100, 114, 115, 119, 123, 136, 140, 153, 174, 175, 176, 185, 195, 206
Heart attack 78
Heart disease 69, 140, 185
Heart weakness. *See* Cardiac insufficiency
Heartburn 118
Hemorrhoids 48, 75, 142, 185
Hepatitis 130, 188
Herbs 18, 26, 70, 85, 89, 98, 102, 121, 143, 168, 169, 195, 213–216
Herbs, wild 18, 26, 70, 85, 102, 195
Herpes 11, 56, 57, 99, 178, 181, 185, 193
HGH. *See* Human growth hormone
High blood pressure 11, 61, 66, 93, 98, 114, 133, 136, 167, 176, 185
Homeopathy 130, 131
Hormones 21, 49, 54, 64, 65, 72, 73, 173

Human Growth Hormone 70
Hunzas 58, 69, 71
Hydrochloric acid 53, 55, 92, 186, 195
Hygiene, Natural. *See* Natural Hygiene

I

Immune system 11, 24, 26, 46, 48, 52, 54, 56, 57, 73, 78, 87, 89, 91, 99, 104, 112, 113, 117, 149, 178, 186, 193
India 40, 113, 116, 131, 136–139, 151, 175–180, 181, 184–190, 193, 195, 197, 198
Indians. *See* Natives
Infection 57, 75, 84, 87, 98, 113, 114, 116–119, 137, 145, 177, 178, 184, 192, 193, 199
Inflammation 75, 115, 116, 121, 138, 169, 175, 176, 178, 186, 187, 188, 195
Injury 56, 63, 93
Intestinal cancer 98
Intestinal Flora 187. *Also see* Flora, intestinal
Intestinal flora 11, 53, 87, 88, 90, 92, 112, 119, 120, 136, 183, 187. *Also see* Flora, intestinal
Intestinal infection 87, 116, 178. *Also see* Colitis
Intestine, large 24
Iron 37, 47, 50, 52

J

Jaundice 142
Joints 21, 124, 176
Joy 3, 13, 19, 21, 24, 26, 29, 51, 54, 77, 84, 140, 154, 205
Juice, fruit 170, 171
Junk food 14, 52

K

Kahunas 40, 143–145, 177, 205
Kelp preparations 190
Kidney 24, 60, 80, 112, 136, 142

L

Laetrile 100, 108
Large intestine 24, 87, 90, 93
Leukemia 106, 145
Libido 54, 71–74, 118, 187
Life expectancy 14, 100
Liver 14, 24, 49, 60, 65, 69, 70, 79, 82, 92, 93, 112, 115, 119, 122–125, 130, 133, 134, 138, 140, 171, 174, 184, 188, 189
Longevity 58, 69, 215
Love 12, 24, 25, 30, 62, 71, 73, 77, 107, 139, 156, 157, 204, 217

Lung cancer 59, 109, 147.
Also see Cancer, lung
Lymph system 145
Lymphocytes 105, 112, 113

M

Magnesium 47, 48, 50, 52, 98, 100, 145
Malaria 131, 138, 188
Massage 76, 80, 84, 151, 152, 153, 158, 188
Maya 150, 219
Meat 27, 38, 39, 58, 77, 82, 83, 88–92, 98, 100, 119, 141, 160, 167, 168, 191, 198, 199, 202
Meat tenderizers 202. *Also see* Tenderizers, meat
Medication 46, 55, 58, 79, 105, 119, 125, 127, 168, 178, 179, 184, 185, 194, 196, 204
Meditation 83, 156, 191
Menopause 72
Menstrual complaints 188
Menstruation 64–67, 179
Metabolism 21, 22, 29, 41, 49, 50, 53, 55, 64, 66, 78, 80–82, 88, 89, 98, 186, 189, 197
Milk 15, 35, 38, 48, 54, 62, 65, 77, 78, 80, 83, 84, 90, 91, 107, 108, 111, 112, 119, 120, 134, 136–139, 141, 143–146, 160, 165, 176, 177, 181, 182, 185, 187, 191, 194, 197, 198, 202
Mind 15, 19, 24–26, 30, 46, 77, 120, 157, 213, 214
Minerals 27, 41, 46–49, 52, 59, 61, 62, 68, 73, 78, 80, 92, 97, 98, 106, 110, 182, 186, 190
Miscarriage 56, 189
Mixed diet 88
MS 57, 98, 189, 211, 212, 217. *Also see* Multiple Sclerosis
Mucous 49, 54, 75, 78, 79, 116–119, 122, 124, 178, 194, 197
Mucous membrane 54, 75, 116, 118, 122, 124, 197
Multiple Sclerosis 57, 189
Multiple sclerosis 113, 116
Muscle pain 49, 146, 189
Muscle paralysis 137, 189
Muscle weakness 50, 137, 152

N

Native Peoples 75, 116, 132, 177
Native peoples 11, 55, 96, 97, 132, 157, 181
Natives of Central and South America 185, 193, 198
Natural Health 94

Natural health 24
Natural Hygiene 25, 27, 29, 47, 96, 97, 98, 112, 140, 204, 208, 213, 214, 218
Nausea 49, 50, 93, 137
Nervous system 65, 66, 75, 79, 83, 142, 173, 178
Nervousness 24, 90, 123, 153
Neurodermatitis 111, 112, 118, 119, 181, 194, 212
Niacin 47, 49
Nicotine 90, 130, 142
Nutrients 72, 88, 97, 100, 101, 119, 149, 154, 173, 187
Nutrition 14, 15, 18, 21, 23, 24, 27, 30, 41, 47, 52, 53, 59, 64, 66, 77, 79, 80–83, 88, 89, 91, 95, 97, 98, 101, 103, 118, 126, 127, 129, 133, 173, 174, 176, 178, 188, 189, 191, 208–211, 211, 213, 215, 218

O

Operations 56, 57, 103, 105, 126, 127, 129, 159, 190
Osteoporosis 21, 48, 50, 80, 167
Overweight 11, 29, 48, 52, 139, 167. *Also see* Reducing weight

P

Pain 23, 28, 48, 49, 57, 79, 84, 103, 113, 119, 124, 126, 127, 128, 129, 131, 132, 134, 137, 140, 142, 145, 146, 187, 189, 193, 195, 220
Pancreas 52, 53, 65, 83, 138, 140, 167, 190
Papain 35, 38, 39, 46, 53–58, 63, 70, 82, 83, 91–95, 103, 104, 107, 112, 115, 116, 124, 125, 128, 130, 137, 138, 143, 150–153, 153, 159, 161, 165, 169–173, 174, 175–197, 202, 203
Parasites 69, 113, 122, 123–125, 130, 134, 138, 142, 143, 171, 182, 190, 196
Pasteurization 62
Pesticides 39, 41, 98, 102, 111
Phosphorus 47, 50
Pineal Gland 65, 184, 191
Pineal gland 65, 130, 184, 191
Pinworms 122, 123, 125, 138
Pituitary gland 65, 90, 121
Poisoning 89, 92, 112, 117. *Also see* Toxins
Potassium 47, 48, 50, 67, 190
Potency 23, 71–74, 128, 131, 187, 211, 214
Powers of self-healing. *See* Self-healing, powers of
Pregnancy 65, 136, 179
Preservatives 90, 97, 102, 165
Prostate 59, 72, 98

221

Protein 18, 33, 47, 49, 50, 51, 53–57, 69, 70, 78, 83, 85, 88, 89, 91–95, 98, 104, 107, 112, 128, 137, 160, 161, 174, 180, 182, 184, 186, 190, 191, 199
Protein digestion 93, 190
Protein supply 191
Psoriasis 117
Purification 112, 192, 213
Putrefying bacteria 83, 88, 92. *Also see* Bacteria, putrefying

R

Raw foods 16, 18, 52, 58, 60, 99, 101, 125, 157, 182, 183. *Also see* Fruit, Vegetable
Raw milk 78, 80
Recipes 66, 110, 130, 132, 136, 146, 148, 152, 157, 158, 160, 161, 167, 175, 202
Recovery 63, 105, 107, 108, 199
Reducing weight 52, 180, 192, 197
Reduction of stress 22, 185
Reiki, Authentic. *See* Authentic Reiki
Rejuvenation 61, 70, 173, 176, 192
Relaxation 25, 26, 83, 142, 185, 208
Remedies 12, 55, 58, 70, 94, 121, 125, 132, 159, 174, 179, 180, 181, 184, 186, 188, 189, 193–196, 198, 213
Rheumatism 22, 28, 57, 80, 82, 99, 113, 116, 124, 126, 141, 145, 167, 173, 193
Riboflavin 47, 49
Rickets 137, 193
Roughage 46, 97, 121
Roundworms 122

S

Salad 58, 59, 69, 72, 78, 153, 160, 161–163, 166, 211, 219
Sattva 12, 29, 140
Seeds 18, 31, 35–41, 42–45, 46, 59, 67, 68, 81, 82, 86, 89, 90, 94, 98, 106, 107, 110–114, 115, 120, 122, 124, 125, 130, 134, 136, 138, 142, 143, 145, 148, 151, 152, 155, 160–162, 164–172, 174, 175, 178–181, 181, 184, 186, 188–194, 194–199, 203
Self-confidence 18, 25, 60, 120
Self-respect 25
Senile speckles 137, 151
Sex 37, 71, 74, 76
Sexually transmitted diseases 193, 197
Shingles 181, 193
Shock 23, 127, 129
Side effects 12, 55–58, 104, 114, 125, 126, 128, 131, 179, 180, 182, 192, 193, 194
Skin 11, 15, 29, 31, 33, 38, 49, 53, 57, 63, 67, 70, 78, 79, 89, 93, 96, 106, 107, 108, 110, 112, 113, 115, 117, 118, 121, 123, 125, 129, 134, 137, 138, 140, 141, 142, 145, 147, 148–153, 161, 167, 169, 170, 178, 179–184, 185, 186, 187, 189, 194, 197, 202, 217
Skin blotches 137
Skin cancer. *See* Cancer, skin
Skin care 150, 202
Sleep 14, 16, 29, 48, 49, 54, 77, 84, 88, 119, 152
Smoking 15, 17, 52, 142
Soil fertility 41
Soil organisms 41, 42
Sore throat 194
Soul 15, 19, 23–25, 26, 29, 120, 140, 157
Spinal injection. *See* Chemonucleolysis
Spirulina 18, 82, 85, 88, 89, 107
Sport 20–21, 56, 58, 64, 194, 197, 219
Sprouts 18, 58, 70, 85, 90, 98, 161
Stomach 23, 28, 48, 82, 89, 92, 93, 102, 113, 116, 119, 120, 125, 132, 134, 138, 142, 146, 153, 157, 171, 186, 191, 193, 195, 196
Stomach ulcers 93
Stomachaches 141
Strength 59, 63, 84, 191, 213
Stress 14, 15, 18, 21, 22, 24–26, 49, 52, 53, 58, 73, 77, 83, 85, 90, 96, 99, 113, 118, 129, 185, 208
Stroke 78, 137, 189
Subtropics 36, 38, 124
Sugar 19, 48, 61, 66, 77, 90, 93, 97, 111, 119, 145, 161, 166, 167, 171
Sun 71, 72, 74, 118, 134, 137, 143, 150–153, 161, 194
Sun food. *See* Food, sun
Sunburn 69, 152, 187, 195
Syphilis 138, 145, 193

T

Tanning 39, 199
Teeth 27, 50, 80, 128, 146, 195
Therapy 30, 39, 54, 55, 56, 57, 62, 70, 79, 83, 84, 100, 101, 102, 103, 104, 105, 106, 107, 108, 109, 114, 116, 118, 127, 129, 133, 136, 151, 154, 170, 173, 174, 175, 176, 177, 178, 179, 182, 184, 185, 187, 189, 193, 194, 197, 199, 203, 210, 211, 212, 214, 215
Thyroid gland 64, 65, 119, 191
Tibetan Rites, Five 15, 23, 26, 129
Tiredness. *See* Chronic fatigue syndrome
Toxemia 66, 96, 97, 112, 140, 211, 218
Travel 123, 156, 161, 196
Treatment, course of 56

Tropics 11, 32, 36, 38, 122–125, 156, 181, 196
Tuberculosis 124, 196
Tumor 57, 79, 95, 105

U

Ulcer 184
Uric acid 82
Uterus 64, 76, 107, 185

V

Varicose veins 11, 23, 48, 56, 190, 197
Vegetable 18, 42, 43, 59–63, 85, 90, 101, 103, 121, 130, 164, 169–173, 173, 188, 211, 212, 219
Vegetable juice 169–173
Vegetarian 15, 18, 99, 101–108, 160, 163, 191, 208, 211, 219
Veins 11, 23, 48, 56, 171, 190, 197
Venereal disease. *See* Sexually transmitted disease
Vermicide 171, 196
Virus 12, 39, 41, 99, 104, 113, 114, 117, 156, 178, 185, 193
Vital components 11, 72, 182
Vitality 14, 63, 84, 88, 91, 102, 211, 213, 217
Vitamin 46–49, 52, 62, 66, 67, 70, 72, 87, 92, 107, 108, 114, 115, 149, 161, 163, 168, 169, 184, 186, 189, 195, 217
Vitamins 15, 27, 41, 46, 47, 52, 53, 59, 60–63, 67, 72, 73, 78, 87, 92, 97, 98, 106, 113, 117, 149, 161, 165, 169, 178, 182, 186, 189
Vomiting 50

W

Warts 134, 137, 141, 152, 181, 197
Weight gain 119
Weight, ideal 16, 28
Weight loss. *See* Reducing weight
Wheat 80, 83, 85, 100, 111, 184, 189, 216
Whipworm 124
WHO 13, 14, 97, 122
Wild herbs. *See* Herbs, wild
World Health Organization. *See* WHO
Worm treatment 171
Worms 93, 113, 122–125, 130, 134, 136, 138, 140, 142, 144, 145, 162, 168, 171, 190, 197, 198

Y

Youth 5, 20, 26, 51, 63, 69, 130, 173, 192

Herbs and other natural health products and information are often available at natural food stores or metaphysical bookstores. If you cannot find what you need locally, you can contact one of the following sources of supply.

Sources of Supply:

The following companies have an extensive selection of useful products and a long track-record of fulfillment. They have natural body care, aromatherapy, flower essences, crystals and tumbled stones, homeopathy, herbal products, vitamins and supplements, videos, books, audio tapes, candles, incense and bulk herbs, teas, massage tools and products and numerous alternative health items across a wide range of categories.

WHOLESALE:

Wholesale suppliers sell to stores and practitioners, not to individual consumers buying for their own personal use. Individual consumers should contact the RETAIL supplier listed below. Wholesale accounts should contact with business name, resale number or practitioner license in order to obtain a wholesale catalog and set up an account.

Lotus Light Enterprises, Inc.
P. O. Box 1008
Silver Lake, WI 531 70 USA
262 889 8501 (phone)
262 889 8591 (fax)
800 548 3824 (toll free order line)

RETAIL:

Retail suppliers provide products by mail order direct to consumers for their personal use. Stores or practitioners should contact the wholesale supplier listed above.

Internatural
33719 116th Street
Twin Lakes, WI 53181 USA
800 643 4221 (toll free order line)
262 889 8581 office phone
WEB SITE: www.internatural.com

Web site includes an extensive annotated catalog of more than 7000 products that can be ordered "on line" for your convenience 24 hours a day, 7 days a week.